i'm THE one PUSHING

A PRACTICAL AND RENEGADE GUIDE TO CHOOSING YOUR OWN MOTHERHOOD ADVENTURE

by

ivette garcía dávila

D1117803

ZINNIA PRESS

LOS ANGELES

This book is nonfiction, though the names and identifying details of people associated with events described in this book may have been changed to protect privacies.

Published by Zinnia Press
3191 Casitas Ave., Ste. 150
Los Angeles, CA 90039

Edited by Jennifer Thomas-Hayes, Beyond Words Editing
Cover Design and Birth Intentions Diagram by Emily Brock
Interior Design by Jennifer Thomas-Hayes and Alessia Vittone

First Edition 2017

ISBN: 978-0-999-01380-9 (Paperback)
        978-0-999-01381-6 (eBook)
LCCN: 2017908596

Note: This book is intended only as a guide for those wishing to know more about pregnancy and motherhood. In no way is this book intended to replace, contradict, or conflict with the advice given to you by your physician. We strongly recommend you follow his or her advice over ours. The author and publisher disclaim all liability in connection with the use of this book and the information it provides.

pH
My love for you is like the universe.

ACKNOWLEDGMENTS

Abigail Morgan
Adrienne McNally
Alan Natali
Alessia Vittone
Alex Elliott
Aimée & Mike Dirksen
Astrid Erismann
Claire & Stephen Broussard
Debbie Torres
Diana Dávila
Emily Brock
Gloria Dávila
Heather Juergensen
Jana Bonderman
Jennifer Thomas-Hayes
Jessica Freeman
Kathleen Dennehy
Kelly & Dan Hauck
Kelly King
Lisa McGuire
Luc Chandou
Maritere Rovira
Matt Miller
Meghann Collins
Nicole West
Nora Dávila
Osmari Fernández
Dr. Patricia Rodriguez Reyes
Ron Forsythe
Sahar Moridani
Sonia Dávila
Sophia Muthuraj
Sydney Poitier
Trina & Brett Jacobsen

SPECIAL THANKS

To my mom, her mom, and her mom's mom:
Ivette María Dávila Casasnovas
Gloria Luisa Casasnovas Alemañy
María Antonia Alemañy Campos

For three generations of strength & kindness.

To my two sisters, and my father and his wife:
Kristina García Dávila
Laura García Dávila
Jose Luis García Villa and Teresa Reyes Reed

For your endless loving support, and because it does take a village.

To my parents-in-law:
Daniel and Cathy Hauck

For showing me a thing or ten about family.

And last, but not least:
To the man who was brave enough to marry me.

Thank you for letting me share.

TABLE OF CONTENTS

~~My Birth Plan~~ *Intentions*   xx

PREFACE: This Book's Conception   xxvii
Incubating a Baby and a Book

1

MY EJACULATE CONCEPTION   1
Baby News Travels...Slowly

A Pregnant Pause   2
Taking In the News

The M-Word   3
Hard Facts About Miscarriage

Safety Advisories (Most) Doctors Agree On   8

Feel Ill?   10
Pregnancy-Safe OTC Medications

Road Map to Prenatal Tests   11
Medical Checkup Timeline

Disseminating the News   16
Creative Ways to Announce Your Pregnancy

Praying for My Vagina and Soul   20
Keep Calm and Carry On

2

WTF HAVE I GOTTEN MYSELF INTO?   21
Birth Your Own "Mamafesto"

Benefits of the Doubt   22
Pushing Through Maternal Insecurity

The Birth of the Mamafesto   23
My Promises to My Daughter

     WRITE YOUR OWN MAMAFESTO   26

3

PRENATAL HEALTH   27
Have Your Cake and Don't Eat It, Too

Perpetuating the Lie   28
Hard-Earned Fitness

Never Say Die-t   29
A Starved Mom = An Unhealthy Baby

Size Matters 30
Eating for One and a Baby

Can and Can't Eats 34

Plating Up 35
Nutritional Needs

Supplementing the Cause 45
Prenatal Vitamins

Read On! 46

Moderation Is Good...in Moderation 47
Permission to Misbehave

Build-A-Snack 48

The Road to Wellville 49
Getting Back to Pre-Pregnancy Glory

4

BRING IT ON, JANE FONDA 51
Keeping Your Pregnant Ass Fit While Your Belly Gets Big

Getting Beat 52
Pregnancy Side Effects

Shake That Pregnant Booty 56
Wiggle It Now, Love It Later

My Favorite Ways to Shake It 57
Pregnancy-Safe Workouts

Pelvic Floor: What, Why, and How? 59

NEAT: Non-Exercise Activity Thermogenesis 61

Other Workouts and Safety Tips   63
Don't Overdo It

Who Let the Farts Out?   66
Know When to Call It Quits

Working Out After Baby   66
Carving Out the Time

5

SEX, LIES, AND MASTURBATE   69
Your Lady Parts Deserve R&R

Pregnant Sex: Safety Guidelines   71
Bumping With a Bump

My *Cosmo*-Worthy Sex Tips   72
Try This at Home

Sex After Baby   74
Working Towards Better Than Ever

6

MY GREEN ALTER-MAMA   77
Baby Steps Towards a Healthier Home and Womb

It Ain't Easy Being Green   78
Trying Is Half the Battle

What Toxins Are in My Home and Womb?   78
Sadly, Lots

The Toxic Table 80

Mr. Green Will See You Now 83
Why Is This Shit Bad for Me and My Baby?

50 Shades of Peroxide 92
Get to the Root of Your Greys

The Tint—and Taint—of Food Dyes 92
What's in a Color?

 To-Dye-For Table 93

Green for Thought 96
Tips for Greenifying Your Life

 GMOS: Superheroes or Supervillains? 97

 The Fluoride in Tap Water Debate 101
 by Heather Juergensen

Sustaining a Green Mindset for the Next Generation 103
Finding Motivation to Be More Hippie-Dippie

Step by Step 104
Pursuing Good Intentions Without Losing Sanity

 Cutout Graphic: Healthy Cheat Sheet 105

7

SERIOUSLY. 107
How Much Crap Does a Teeny-Weeny Little Baby Need?

Baby List & Registry 109
Junior's Bounty

Baby Registry Confidential 109
Keeping It Real on Your Shopping Spree

List o' Crap and Goodies You May (or May Not) Need   113
Baby Gear from A to Z

     Diaper Bag Survival Kit   136

Baby Shower Confidential   151
The Politics of Parties

8

LABOR A LA CARTA   155

Eeny, Meeny, Miny, Moe...Mi Mamá Picks the Very Best One

Birth 101: Attend or Cut Class?   156
Prepping for the Mother of All Tests

To Push or Not to Push?   157
Hopefully, You Get to Decide

     Some Questions to Consider When Your Doctor Says:
     "Let's Get This Baby Out of Here"   158
     by Abigail Morgan, LAc, FABORM

     Tears Over Tears   161

     Enjoying the C-Ride (the Second Time Around)   164
     by Adrienne M.

     What to Expect When You're Not Expecting   168
     by Kathleen Dennehy

Where Should I Have My Baby?   169
Hospital, Birthing Center, Home, or Minivan

     Pain Med Dessert Menu   170

     Enjoying a Drug-Free Birth (the Second Time Around)   172
     by Maritere Rovira Calimano

     My Hospital Bill   176

What's an Episiotomy? — 178

Perineal Massage — 179

Birthing Woes — 180

Signs of Labor — 182

Backseat Baby — 183
by Alex Elliott

To Doula or Not to Doula? — 189
Finding Your Doulmate

Do I Bank That Cord? — 191
Save It, Share It, or Toss It

Do I Keep Baby Connected to the Mother "Landline"? — 193
Placental Transfusion

WTF Is Apgar? — 194

Placenta Smoothie, *Por Favor* — 194
Consume Your Own Goods...or Not

Do I Give Baby Erythromycin? — 195
Eyes Wide Shut

Vitamin K...Krazy or Kool? — 196
Why You Might Give It a Shot

Circumspect About Circumcision? — 197
Deciding Whether to Make the Cut

Map Your Own Adventure — 199
As Much As Fate Allows...

My Birth ~~Plan~~ Intentions — 200

9

WE MAKE PLANS AND GOD LAUGHS AT OUR VAGINAS

205

My Birthing Story: A Page-One Rewrite

"You Can't Always Get What You Want" **205**
Labor Induction

    The Lowdown on Pitocin   **208**

I'm the One Pushing...Right? **212**
Taking Charge of Labor

Pushed, Unsealed, Delivered...I'm Yours! **214**
"You Get What You Need"

The Final Insult **215**
Wait a Minute—We Have to Go Back In

Confessions of a Happy Mom **216**
Coulda, Shoulda, Woulda...But Who Cares?

    Chronology of My Induced Labor   **217**

    SAT-Worthy Labor Vocabulary   **218**

10

BRINGING UP BABY

221

Who Invited the Peanut Gallery?

Mother (-in-Law) Knows Best **223**
We Ain't Got This

It Takes a Village, and There's Always an Idiot (Me)   **226**
Family Intervention

Don't Sleep When She Sleeps   **230**
Find Your Saving Grace

If You Can Afford It, Pay for It   **231**
Budgeting Me-Time

A Love Triangle   **232**
Romancing After Baby

"What's Love Got to Do With It?"   **238**
Realistically Ever After

11

TO VACCINATE OR NOT TO VACCINATE?   241
Is There a Question?

Anti-Vaccine Arguments   **241**
Diving Deep into Claims

Vaccine Side Effects   **243**
Risk and Benefit Analysis

Herd Immunity   **244**
Disease-Free Utopia

Stats Speak Louder Than Words   **245**
Vaccine Efficacy, Disputed Ingredients, and Safety Testing

Challenging the Middle Ground   **248**
Making Educated Decisions

The Bottom Line   249
The Impact of Your Choice

12

SICK IS A FOUR-LETTER WORD   253
Fussing Over a Fussy Baby

The Unlucky Seven   254
From Mom to Mom, Baby's Sickness Handbook

    Taking the Temp on Thermometer Choices   257

Homeopathic Schomeopathic...*Abuelita en la Casa!*   266
Grandma's Natural Remedies

    Essential Oils: DYI Healing Blends   269
    by Claire Chandou Broussard

Over-the-Counter Pain & Fever Reducers   273
What's in a Medicine?

Anti-Antibiotics   275
Fighting the Resistance

    What I Wish I Would've Known About MRSA   276
    by Jessica Racioppo Freeman

In Doc We Trust   278
But Still, Follow Your Gut

    Read On!   279

13

BREASTFEEDING SUCKS 281

Pumping's Just Another Word for Nothing Left to Lose

Pro-Choice 282
Formula Is Okay. Really.

A Double-Edged Boob 284
When Baby Only Drinks from Tata

    Push Tips for the Breastfeeding Mama 286

The Grass Is Always Greener 288
Playing a Good Hand With the Breasts You're Dealt

How I Learned to Stop Sobbing and Love the Boob 288
Embracing the Milking of Ivette García Dávila

Breast Is, in Most Cases, Best 289
But Only If Good for Mom

TRUTH OR STRETCH?
Debunking Some Tata-Juice Myths 290
It's Not a Panacea—But It Does Have Perks

    SIDS: Minimizing the Risk 294

Love in the Time of Formula 298
Finding the Best for Baby

    What Is a Supplemental Nursing System? 300

Did I Say Breastfeeding Sucks?
I Must Not Have Pumped Much. 302
The Pain and Practicality of Pumping

    Push Tips for the Pumping Mama 305

BUI: Breastfeeding Under the Influence   306
Drink Smarter, Not Harder

14

THE BABY, THE BOSS, THE HOME, & YOUR LOVER   311
Juggling Life While Exclusively Breastfeeding

State of the Union: Maternity Leave   312
Cobbling Together Baby-Bonding Time

    Maternity Leave Laws   312

Milked Dry   313
Breastfeeding 9 to 5

Dropping the Ball   315
Being a Good Juggler Isn't Everything

A Mother in the Modern World   316
What's in a Mom?

In Pursuit of Happiness   321
Permission to Pursue Your Dreams

15

DOGGED MOMMY GUILT   323
Bite It Before It Bites You

The Blame Game   326
Facing Down Mommy Issues

Guilt: Do Not Recycle   328
The Art of Self-Forgiveness

Debunking the Marth   330
Managing Expectations

Practice Makes Imperfect   331
"I'm Not Like Them, but I Can Pretend"

AFTERWORD: Postpartum Reflections   335
The Good, the Bad, and the Awesome

The Fear Parasite   335
Love Hurts

The End of an Era   337
Fighting the Stereotype

The New Cool   340
Mom Is the New Black

Me, the Mom   341
Applying My Motherhood Skills to Life

Me, the Human Being   343
Breaking Out of the Mom Mold

Me, the Wife   344
It's Okay to Forget About Your Kid Sometimes

Oh, Shit (and Other Joys of Motherhood)   346
The Adventure of a Lifetime

BIBLIOGRAPHY   351

My Birth

I want

- NATURAL LABOR
- VBAC
- ELECTIVE C-SECTION
- NON-ELECTIVE C-SECTION

HOME

Birth CENTER

+ Hospital

Water Birth

PLEASE

LET ME MOVE AROUND THE HOSPITAL ROOM

KEEP ME IN BED & MONITOR BABY & MAMA

DRUGS

NO

PLEASE + PRONTO

NOT SURE—WILL DECIDE WHEN I FEEL LIKE IT

IF MY BABY IS LATE

PLEASE WAIT

VISIT ACUPUNCTURIST

INDUCE

BREAK MY WATER

CERVICAL RIPENING

PITOCIN

IF COMPLICATIONS ARISE DURING MY NATURAL LABOR

ONCE DELIVERED, IF BABY IS HEALTHY, I WANT BABY

TAKE ME TO THE OR & GIVE ME A C-SECTION!

LET ME CONSULT/ GET 2ND OPINION

IN MY ROOM AT ALL TIMES

GIVE ME TIME... I MAY GET THERE

LET ME KISS MY LOVER FOR GOOD LUCK

IN THE NURSERY (I WANT TO REST)

~~PLAN~~ INTENTIONS

I WANT TO LISTEN/WATCH

QUIET   MUSIC   TV   CONVERSATIONS

shh!

TOP 3 PLAYLIST:

1:

2:

3:

FAVORITE
SHOW:

I WANT

DARK OR LOW LIGHT

SUN—BASK IN NATURAL LIGHT IF POSSIBLE

CANDLES

    SCENTED

    UNSCENTED

MY GUEST LIST

1.

   (MY LABOR PARTNER/ADVOCATE)

2.

3.

4.

5.

6.

Chill to TOAST after baby →

my Rules ↓

1.

2.

3.

4.

5.

6. FEED ME:

IN MY DELIVERY BAG

1.

2.

3.

4.

5.

NO

ALLOWED, PLEASE!

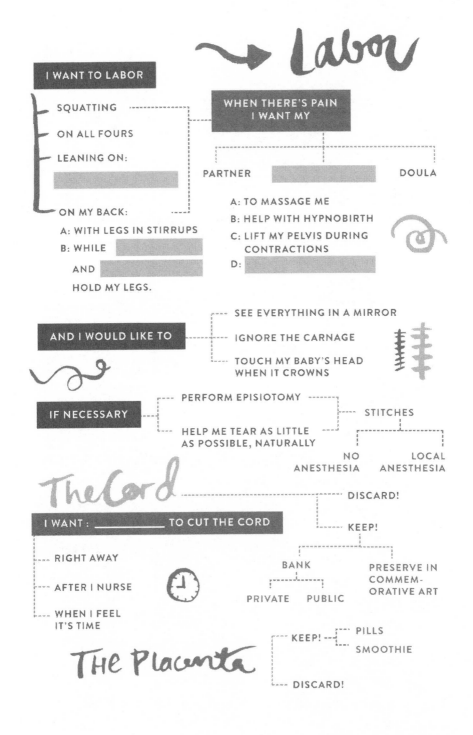

Labor

I WANT TO LABOR

- SQUATTING
- ON ALL FOURS
- LEANING ON: [   ]
- ON MY BACK:
    - A: WITH LEGS IN STIRRUPS
    - B: WHILE [   ]
      AND [   ]
      HOLD MY LEGS.

WHEN THERE'S PAIN I WANT MY

PARTNER   [   ]   DOULA

- A: TO MASSAGE ME
- B: HELP WITH HYPNOBIRTH
- C: LIFT MY PELVIS DURING CONTRACTIONS
- D: [   ]

AND I WOULD LIKE TO

- SEE EVERYTHING IN A MIRROR
- IGNORE THE CARNAGE
- TOUCH MY BABY'S HEAD WHEN IT CROWNS

IF NECESSARY

- PERFORM EPISIOTOMY
- HELP ME TEAR AS LITTLE AS POSSIBLE, NATURALLY

STITCHES
- NO ANESTHESIA
- LOCAL ANESTHESIA

The Cord

I WANT : _____ TO CUT THE CORD

- RIGHT AWAY
- AFTER I NURSE
- WHEN I FEEL IT'S TIME

- DISCARD!
- KEEP!
    - BANK
        - PRIVATE
        - PUBLIC
    - PRESERVE IN COMMEMORATIVE ART

The Placenta

- KEEP!
    - PILLS
    - SMOOTHIE
- DISCARD!

For my Baby

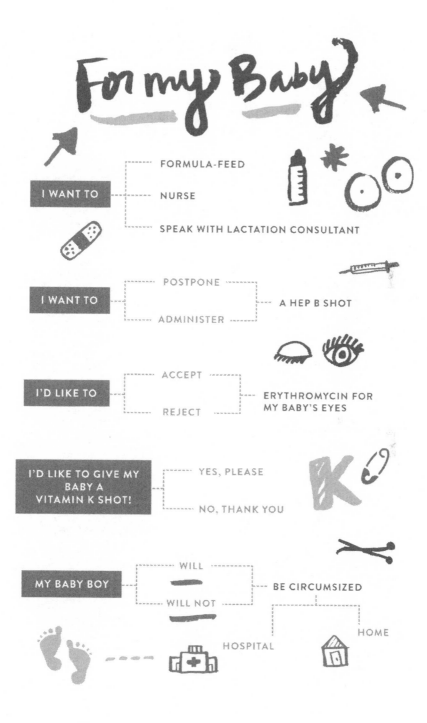

I WANT TO
- FORMULA-FEED
- NURSE
- SPEAK WITH LACTATION CONSULTANT

I WANT TO
- POSTPONE
- ADMINISTER

A HEP B SHOT

I'D LIKE TO
- ACCEPT
- REJECT

ERYTHROMYCIN FOR MY BABY'S EYES

I'D LIKE TO GIVE MY BABY A VITAMIN K SHOT!
- YES, PLEASE
- NO, THANK YOU

MY BABY BOY
- WILL
- WILL NOT

BE CIRCUMSIZED

HOSPITAL

HOME

i'm the one PUSHING

PREFACE:

THIS BOOK'S CONCEPTION

Incubating a Baby and a Book

BEFORE I GOT PREGNANT, I knew very little about prenatal care, giving birth, and newborn safekeeping. When a pregnant friend texted me: *Braxton Hicks are such a pain,* I thought she had mistyped "kicks" and that her baby would be named Braxton! She still makes fun of me for not knowing she was referring to the false labor contractions women sometimes suffer prior to the real deal.

And motherhood? Well, I was ill-prepared, to say the least. So I sought out information that would help me take on pregnancy and being a mom.

First, I turned to books. Most of them were either full of important information but long and dull and *too* specific, or packed with irreverent humor but lacking the all-encompassing practical advice a first-time mother needs. I wanted a comprehensive book that was entertaining enough to tickle my funny bone yet sufficiently fact-balanced to indulge my brain noodle. I didn't have the time to read through ten library tomes. But I ended up reading all of them trying to find *the* one.

It didn't exist.

I couldn't find a single book that discussed all the alternatives that were overwhelming me and would help me make educated decisions. A book that felt *real* and could walk me from conception through pregnancy nutrition, fitness, preparing a healthy home, making a registry, birthing my baby, caring for her, breastfeeding, going back to work, and coping with motherhood—plus provide some emotional support and laughs to boot. The few books that covered some of these topics together felt dated, impersonal, disingenuous, a little scary, or, at times, one-sided.

I wasn't the sort of mom-to-be who adored being pregnant; I wasn't particularly interested in reveling in the magic of childbirth. I was simply eager to survive it all because I wanted a child so very badly. Some books made me feel inadequate because I felt disconnected with that aspect of motherhood. I wanted straightforward information that allowed me to make up my own mind about (a) how to best care for my body and baby while pregnant, (b) what sort of labor was best suited for me, and (c) most importantly, what kind of mother I wanted to be. I wanted to learn how to juggle motherhood and still remain "me."

While trying to equip myself with knowledge through books and the Internet, everyone and their mothers barraged me with old wives' tales, denouncement or praise for popular trends, and their own understanding of maternal expectations in society. If I had to hear one more time: "When you're a mother, you won't be able to _____ [insert any verb you enjoy doing here, like 'vacation' or 'drink a lot']," I was gonna push this baby out and give her to the wolves. They would at least provide a simple and clear path into adulthood.

So much of what I was told sounded questionable or just didn't feel right for *me*. Sure, my mom and mom-in-law eagerly imparted a wealth of valuable knowledge. But some of their intel was outdated. They didn't know about current baby gadgetry or what types of exercises were safe to do while pregnant. They didn't know about recent nutritional and environmental findings, or answers to questions like *Is breastmilk really all that much better than formula?* Plus, I had questions about sex and stuff, and I wasn't about to ask *them* if doggie-style could take me through the last trimester.

I wanted to dig into the detailed truth behind all the blanket advice.

My lifelong friends who'd had babies young also taught me a lot. But having given birth a decade ago, they still thought "pumping and dumping" was a great way to booze it up while breastfeeding. And although my contemporary mom friends who were also pushing forty (and babies) *did* know about current standards, I worried about sounding stupid or about things getting weird when my opinions clashed with theirs. *No TV 'til they're two? Really?* Shit, I already had old-school *Sesame Street* downloaded onto our iPad. And the big one: *What about vaccines?* There are so many divisive topics in the mom community.

I felt like I was lost inside a creepy funhouse trying to find my way out, or at least flip on a light switch so I could make sense of my own distorted reflection. Every mirror reflected me differently. Just like each of the choices that lay ahead outlined a different kind of mom. *Which mom was I?*

I was determined to find my way.

I became a student. I took notes on everything I learned through reading, talking to hundreds of mothers, and from my own mistakes. What I ended up with was a part-guide, part-memoir journal full of well-researched material, other mothers' testimonials, and my own discoveries about pregnancy, labor, and those first years of motherhood, which sometimes defied traditional conventions. Things like: you can still have great sex even after stretching your vagina to the circumference of your baby's head (and shoulders), that with a little work your body can bounce back to (a notch below) its former glory, and that life "as you know it" doesn't have to be (totally) over.

I decided to turn my revelations into the book I would have wanted to read before I even got pregnant, so I could share it with other like-minded women. Practical moms-to-be who are sensible and realistic about the "magic" of it all. Healthy moms in need of nurturing their own identities as well as their children's. Chicks who don't mind blazing a trail if the outlined path feels too trodden. Renegade girls who feel like a cow in a china shop at PTA meetings, resist being *just* a mom, or rush bedtime because they can't wait to pop open a bottle of wine. We don't have to be the mom everyone thinks we ought to be. Like soldiers, we moms need to be all we *can* be. And that's hard enough as it is.

As a new mom, I faced parental hardships others had warned me about but I didn't believe, plus other things I didn't even know would be a "thing."

Things like how much breastfeeding can suck, or how much a newborn really shits, or how much you'll really miss being alone, or the fear parasite that lives off the omnipresent love you feel for your child.

Some days you'll wake up and wish you could call in sick and be excused from all motherhood duties. You'll show up to "work" in a shitty mood and plop your kid in front of your go-to sitter, Peppa Pig. It's okay to feel that way. You're a woman who has a purpose in life, and sometimes your kid gets in the way—no need to feel guilt over that. Other times, your baby will giggle or say "Mama" in a sweet singsong voice dripping with love and admiration, and you'll whisper in her tiny ear: "I was put on this earth to be your mom." Both sentiments are natural and not mutually exclusive. Motherhood is very yin and yang.

I'm the One Pushing doesn't pretend to have it all or know it all. It's merely a companion piece to your own motherhood adventure. In my journey, I started out a bit overconfident, thinking I was gonna "kill it." After all, I had done my research. Boy, was I wrong! The cocky woman who started writing this book is not the reflective mother who finished it. Because I wrote it in chronological order, you'll see what motherhood did to me. And I mean this in the best possible way. Like most mothers, I'm just an ordinary gal trying to do something extraordinary: raise another human being without downgrading my own human status. It's a war we moms fight every day, and sometimes we lose the day's battle. But it's *our* war and nobody else's.

Whether you decide to push without drugs in a tub while someone rubs your clitoris (it's a thing); adopt a baby; put your eggs in someone else's basket; sign up for an epidural nine months in advance; schedule a C-section for medical reasons *or* because you're too posh to push like V. Beckham—it's solely your own business what, why, and how you do this mom thing every step of the way. You can tell everyone else to go push a baby out of their own vagina. Or penis.

You're the one pushing. Or having a C-section. Or picking up your baby in Ethiopia. Not every mom carries her baby in her womb, but in my book, *all* moms are pushers. If you're looking to adopt or find a surrogate, you may still find the information in this book helpful, especially if you'll be involved with the birth mother's labor.

Of course, no book can totally prepare a mother for the journey that lies ahead. I only hope my experiences can help you forge your own path and equip you with enough knowhow and humor to survive becoming a mother and the first few roller-coaster years of raising a child. Take my advice—and everyone else's—with a mine of salt. As if you were chasing tequila.

Choose your own Mom-venture.

Ivette Garcia Davila

MY EJACULATE CONCEPTION

Baby News Travels...Slowly

THE PEE STICK said I wasn't pregnant. I didn't believe it. Underneath my plaid miniskirt, I could feel an embryo growing on my sexy uterine lining. But I shrugged it off. *I guess I can keep drinking,* I consoled myself as I fastened my stripper Mary Janes to complete my Catholic schoolgirl Halloween costume.

Don't judge me. I had nothing else to dress up as.

Six days later, still no period. So I peed on a stick again. I watched the pregnancy test intently, waiting for the parallel lines to become sharp as I wiped piss off my fingers. Way more fun than watching paint dry.

I'd dreamed about those two lines indicating a positive result for years. And at last, my wish came true! I was finally not not-pregnant after six weeks of not not-trying. Two negatives making a positive—I knew my algebra-teacher mother would be proud.

I went out for my daily hike on a warm Los Angeles "fall" morning. I wanted to walk the earth being the only person in it knowing I was with child. Plus, I had to figure out how to tell the father of this unborn baby—the hesitant ejaculator in our premeditated unprotected sexual experience that had led to this semi-planned pregnancy.

1

I had wanted to get pregnant and my husband had finally agreed to stop using contraceptives, thinking it would take a while. A baseball fanatic, I hope he now appreciates that he hit a homerun in the first inning. It probably helped that sneaky me stuck in a tampon after sex to improve our odds. But we won't tell him that. His "boys" get all the credit.

I felt grateful and guilty all at once. I had heard from some of my friends how difficult, frustrating, and emotionally draining it had been for them to get pregnant—taking hormones, tracking cycles, monitoring egg temperatures, taking Chinese herbs, doing acupuncture, even undergoing a few rounds of in vitro fertilization (IVF). And here we were, two rookies who had just hit a grand slam—though strictly speaking, that would have meant we were having triplets. Thankfully, this was a single. I was barely ready for one. He was barely ready for none. And I had to break the news.

A Pregnant Pause

I found my husband by our little-engine-that-could air conditioner in the corner of our bedroom. I walked up to him, all stinky after my hike.

"I'm pregnant," I blurted (no exclamation point). The air conditioner breathed loudly, evaporating the sweat off my skin but leaving the stickiness behind.

My husband kissed the top of my head (or was it my forehead?) and murmured something neither of us can remember. Something like "Holy shit" or "You're fucking pregnant." No exclamation point on either.

It took him a while to process his impending fatherhood. Our unborn daughter became the elephant baby in the room for the next few weeks. But soon, his love for our daughter and joy over becoming a dad began (and continues) to grow every single day.

I, on the other hand, felt like the star in my own musical from day one. I had wanted to be a mom since I'd cradled my first Cabbage

Patch Kid. Since then, I'd imagined a toddler running into my open arms; heart-to-hearts cuddled under a blanket lit by a flashlight; watching my favorite childhood movies together: *Girls Just Want to Have Fun* and *The Little Mermaid;* picking up seashells and returning them to the ocean; whispering tiny secrets and big ones; crying and laughing over a serious and silly life.

It took a supersized serving of self-control not to break in song and dance during that epic first post-pregnant hike and the weeks that followed as I kept the suggested vow of silence. It's recommended you wait until week 12 to reveal the news of your pregnancy, due to the risk of miscarriage in the first trimester.

The M-Word

Call it beginner's luck (or sheer naiveté), but in spite of being thirty-five and entering the "advanced maternal age" bracket, I embraced a positive outlook about my pregnancy early on. And I was comforted by the overall odds: The majority of pregnancies do end in a live birth.

However and unfortunately, miscarriages are common during the first twelve weeks—especially the first eight. In fact, many women miscarry before they even know they're pregnant. Which is why, unless you're going through intrauterine insemination (IUI) or IVF, or you need to track the first signs of pregnancy for medical reasons, it's recommended to avoid taking early pregnancy tests. A pregnancy can dissolve itself before the next period arrives and "ignorance is bliss" may be a good way to live.

Even armed with all the positive vibes in the world, it's hard not to worry about miscarriage when you're already head over heels in love with the baby in your belly. Suffering a miscarriage is one of the biggest fears (if not THE biggest fear) women face during pregnancy.

The statistics presented here will hopefully allow you to remain at least cautiously optimistic during the first trimester.

WHAT'S A MISCARRIAGE?

Miscarriage (or spontaneous abortion) is the medical term for embryo or fetal loss during the first twenty weeks of pregnancy. Usually, the body discharges the lost fetus, but sometimes a dilation and curettage (D&C) procedure is necessary to clear the uterus lining, especially if miscarriage occurs towards the end of the twenty-week window.

HARD FACTS ABOUT MISCARRIAGE

- For most women, miscarriage happens only once in a lifetime.

- Although some findings indicate otherwise, a recent comprehensive study found that women who'd suffered a previous miscarriage did not have a significantly higher risk of miscarriage than those who hadn't.

- Between 10 and 20 percent of pregnancies end in miscarriage, which means 80 to 90 percent end in live births.

- A full 80 percent of miscarriages occur in the first twelve weeks; hence, the chances for a healthy baby look good once you've completed the first trimester.

- In the first trimester, the risk of miscarriage decreases as you go, so your odds improve daily as you close in on the twelve-week mark.

- The risk of losing a pregnancy after twelve weeks is only 2 to 4 percent.

- Between 50 and 70 percent of miscarriages are due to chromosome abnormalities.

- Women with history of vaginal bleeding in pregnancy (as opposed to just spotting or discharge) are 2.6 times likelier to miscarry.

- Cigarette smoking increases the odds of miscarriage.

- Nausea and vomiting (NVP, a.k.a. morning sickness) during the first trimester usually indicates a healthy placenta, which would mean a lower risk of miscarriage and preterm labor. Nausea alone is linked to a 50 percent reduction in risk, while vomiting is linked to a 75 percent reduction. But don't panic: I, along with many women I know, remained immune to morning sickness and went on to have perfectly healthy babies. BTW, the term "morning sickness" needs to be modified to "around-the-clock sickness," according to my friends who did suffer from it (and also went on to have healthy babies).

- The detection of a heartbeat corresponds to dramatically lowered chances of a miscarriage. Therefore, once you've confirmed cardiac activity, your own heart can beat a little steadier.

- Miscarriage risk increases gradually after Mom is age thirty-five and spikes after age forty. In a study of 2,139 women, the miscarriage rate after confirmation of fetal viability was 14 percent in those ages forty and up, versus 2 percent for those thirty-nine and under.

- Dad's age also has a negative effect, especially after he passes age forty.

WHY DO MISCARRIAGES HAPPEN?

As much as we'd love to pinpoint an exact cause, some miscarriages are simply medically unexplainable or are difficult to be studied for a myriad of reasons, including that most of them happen at home.

According to the American Pregnancy Association (APA), the most common cause of miscarriage is chromosomal abnormalities.

Chromosomal abnormalities can occur during cell division as the embryo is forming. A cell may split unevenly and/or genetic information may be lost or triplicated, which can sometimes result in a miscarriage.

Abnormalities can also occur through genetics. However, unless both parents pass on an abnormal gene onto the zygote (fertilized ovum) upon conception, most gene abnormalities don't result in fetal abnormality. If one half of the chromosomal pair is healthy, in most cases, it takes over the "set." Genetics are fascinating.

Miscarriage Warning Signs

Call your doctor or midwife immediately if you suffer from any of these symptoms:

- Very strong cramps at fixed intervals, resembling contractions.

- Heavy brown or red bleeding.

- Thick, grayish tissue-like discharge.

- Spotting or bleeding during the second trimester. (Note: It is not unusual for bleeding and cramps to occur after sexual activity, though it is still always wise to ring the doctor.)

More encouraging words: A friend of mine had fairly heavy unexplained bleeding during her second trimester. She carried to term and gave birth to a beautiful baby girl.

Why some babies with chromosomal abnormalities make it out of the womb and others don't is greatly disputed. Some think that the mother's immune system "attacks" the anomalous pregnancy while others think that the chromosomal abnormalities prevent the fetus from developing. Regardless, for better or worse, most babies with abnormalities don't make it out of the womb.

A smaller risk of miscarriage is accounted for by any of the following: listeria, maternal hormonal or structural abnormalities, injury or abdominal trauma (such as falling on your stomach), age, disease, infection, chronic illness.

If you do suffer this loss, don't be ashamed and do not feel guilty.

CAN MISCARRIAGES BE PREVENTED?

A mother who takes care of herself is never at fault for a miscarriage or a fetal abnormality. Treating your pregnant body well, taking supplements, maximizing quality of life, minimizing stress and toxins, heeding your doctor's precautions, and abstaining from restricted behaviors is *all* you can do to ensure that your baby has the best chance not only inside the womb but outside of it. Having a daily cup of coffee, exercising moderately, or having sex will not harm your baby. And, debatably (see textbox on next page), an occasional glass of wine after the first trimester is fine; but proceed with caution: Fetal alcohol spectrum disorders (FASD) *are* a real thing and 100 percent preventable.

There's nothing you can do to alter the genetic factors set in place at conception. However, in certain situations, if a risk assessment dictates it and the process is carefully monitored, medical techniques can be used to try to avoid miscarriage.

Because low progesterone has been associated with miscarriage, a few studies indicate that taking progesterone could lessen the risk of miscarriage in women who have a history of miscarrying. Progesterone is also used to avoid miscarriage in women using reproductive technologies such as IVF. At the time of this book's publishing, not enough evidence has been compiled to suggest that taking progesterone supplements could help a woman without any previous miscarriages who got pregnant the old-fashioned way; but that's not to say it's impossible.

Baby aspirin could also help prevent miscarriages in women with a history of miscarriage or who have a blood disorder, such as thrombophilia. The theory is that because aspirin can act as a blood thinner, it can prevent blood clots and help blood get into the placenta. **Please do note that using aspirin during pregnancy must be cleared by a doctor.** Aspirin, even in low doses, can cause serious complications.

BIG NO-NO!

Safety Advisories (Most) Doctors Agree On

- Don't take a hot bath (your body temperature needs to stay under 102 degrees).

- Don't get X-rays.

- Don't smoke.

- Don't do drugs intended for Burning Man.

- Don't drink during the first trimester, or excessively at any point in your pregnancy.*

*A survey conducted in 2010 reported that 66 percent of OB/GYNs recommend not drinking at all during pregnancy, whereas 34 percent agree with the Royal College of Obstetricians and Gynecologists that occasional alcohol intake hasn't been proven to be harmful to fetuses. I went with the Royals on this one.

Don't Freak Out If...

Every pregnancy is different, and yours may well be more difficult than those of your friends. Universally, all of the following symptoms are completely normal during pregnancy. However, always consult your doctor if you feel a side effect is happening too often and/or affecting your well-being.

Spotting. One-third of pregnant women spot during the first trimester. When experiencing light spotting, sex and exercise should be avoided.

Mild lower-back pain and cramps. This type of pain, resembling menstrual cramps, is also common in the first trimester. A heating pad on your lower back may help ease pain and it won't hurt your baby. But do not apply heat to your abdomen.

Breast tenderness. Hormonal shifts cause a spike in blood volume and changes in breast tissue, which results in sore boobs. I found wearing a sports bra comfy during this stage.

Headaches. These can be due to a variety of causes, from hormones to changes in blood flow to posture and weight gain, to stress, poor sleep, and/or caffeine withdrawl. The list goes on!

Vaginal discharge. This is also in the pregnancy "garden variety." Your lady parts are working to keep a thriving cervix, which often manifests in white gunk in your underwear.

Dr. Jekyll and Mrs. Hyde Syndrome. Your emotional highs and lows may be so diametrically opposed, you'll need a new metric system just to keep tabs on your mood swings. There's not much you can do about this except remind those around you that they're much loved and explain to them how little control you have over your hormones.

Feel Ill?

Being pregnant and sick at the same time can feel like a double-whammy. By no means should you suffer without seeking some medicinal relief, but there are some precautions to heed. Most OTC medications do cross the placenta, and a fetus is most susceptible during the first trimester.

Avoid products with Bismuth subsalicylate (think Pepto Bismol) or Atropine/diphenoxylate (Lomotil).

Unless your doctor advises against it, it is usually safe to take recommended doses of the following medications for a few days during pregnancy:

Advil *	Maalox
Benadryl	Metamucil
Claritin	Senokot
Colace	Tamiflu
Dulcolax	Zantac
Imodium A-D	steroid nasal sprays
Kaopectate	most cough drops

except during the third trimester

BIG NØ-NØ!
Tylenol is not recommended for pregnant women, as it has been linked with a higher rate of asthma in their children.

Some studies also suggest pregnant women avoid medications with the expectorant guaifenesin (e.g., Mucinex), the decongestant pseudoephedrine (e.g., Sudafed), or the cough suppressant dextromethorphan (e.g., Benylin DM), although they are generally considered safe.

If you are braving a bad one (been there), choose a medication that targets your specific symptoms instead of an all-in-one so that you don't take unnecessary drugs. It's also wise to steer clear of nighttime medications and cough syrups, as they may contain alcohol.

Finally, you might want to consider natural remedies, which we discuss in *Chapter 12: Sick Is a Four-Letter Word.*

BOTTOM LINE

There are many ways to combat the worries that plague us during pregnancy and, later on, motherhood. Exercise, meditation, and religion come to mind. But above all, try to stay in the present and enjoy this time of calm before the storm! Find a doctor you trust (and like), and put yourself in her hands—you'll be seeing her a lot in the next nine months.

Road Map to Prenatal Tests

Long before ultrasounds and fancy blood screens, people managed to bring healthy babies into this world. However, thanks to modern medicine, we're able to obtain information that can help us monitor potential problems and make game-changing decisions during our pregnancy.

Below is a general outline of doctor's visits and testing performed for a standard pregnancy. Having this list helped me feel informed during my appointments, able to ask such questions as: "Are my progesterone levels okay?" or "How is my baby's neck looking?" I hope this guide helps you navigate your own prenatal-care course.

PRENATAL CHECKUP TIMELINE

6–9 Weeks

Physical exam: This may include a breast, pap, and pelvic exam, depending on how long it's been since your previous checkup.

Ultrasound: To evaluate the presence of fetal heart activity and/or establish gestational age.

Urine screen: Some doctors require samples every time you visit, to monitor various levels (such as human chorionic gonadotropin [hCG], the hormone produced by the placenta after implantation). Luckily, since you're pregnant, peeing shouldn't be a big deal. Now, the aiming into the cup part...

Blood screen: If it's your first pregnancy or you're visiting a new health practice, you may need a blood test to determine your blood group and establish whether you're Rh-positive or negative. Blood may also be used for other standard prenatal tests, such as detecting congenital genetic disorders, checking thyroid function, and monitoring progesterone levels. You can also request a check of your vitamin D, lead, and mercury levels.

9–14 Weeks

First trimester ultrasound or nuchal translucency scan (NT scan): This ultrasound measures the fluid buildup at the back of your baby's neck. The liquid appearing thick could be an indication (but not a diagnosis) of chromosomal abnormalities, or conditions such as Noonan syndrome. This ultrasound may also catch signs of cardiovascular problems.

Non-invasive prenatal testing (NIPT): Depending on your age and medical history, your doctor may recommend a blood screen to check for chromosomal abnormalities. This test may also detect the sex of baby. Note that, unlike the quad screen (detailed below), it does not evaluate placental dysfunction or other risk factors. If you're over thirty-five or have relevant medical history, it's likely your insurance will at least partially cover this test.

If either of the aforementioned tests comes back with a possibility of chromosomal abnormality or cardiovascular issues, you can request an early CVS during this period. More information on that test below.

14–19 Weeks

Quadruple screen ("quad screen") a.k.a. multiple marker: A non-invasive integrated blood screen that can identify neural tube defects (NTD) and foresee placental complications. This can help determine your risk of preterm delivery, fetal growth restriction, placental abruption, intrauterine fetal demise, or preeclampsia. Though not as accurate as the NIPT in detecting signs of chromosomal abnormalities, it does screen for them. A positive result would indicate a need for further testing.

Amniocentesis: An optional procedure in which a needle is inserted into the uterus through the abdomen to withdraw a small sample of amniotic fluid. The fluid is examined for genetic abnormalities such as Down's Syndrome (a.k.a. trisomy 21) or Edward's Syndrome (a.k.a. trisomy 18). This test is also recommended to women with a high risk of having a baby with NTD, as it has a 95 percent detection rate. This procedure may slightly increase chances of miscarriage.

Chorionic villus sampling (CVS): This optional test is performed in lieu of amniocentesis to detect chromosomal abnormalities and other conditions. A CVS examines chorionic villus cells retrieved from the placenta at the spot where it connects to the uterine wall. The most common way to biopsy the developing placenta is through the cervix, but it's also collected transabdominally (like amniocentesis).

Unlike amniocentesis, a CVS can be performed early, during weeks 10–13, which is useful for high-risk patients. The risk of miscarriage after this procedure is similar to that of amniocentesis, or perhaps a little higher.

20–22 Weeks

Structural ultrasound or fetal morphology a.k.a. anomaly scan: A non-invasive abdominal ultrasound performed by a perinatologist, which measures your baby's limbs, organs, and bones. This test may help detect anencephaly (absence of the top of the head), hydrocephalus (excess fluid in the brain), cleft lip, abdominal wall defects, kidney issues, major heart problems, and some chromosomal abnormalities.

24–28 Weeks

Diabetes screening: A one-hour glucose test that involves drinking an awful syrupy substance that tastes like two-day-old Fanta and then getting your blood drawn exactly one hour afterward. This is to check Mom for gestational diabetes. Only 2–5 percent of women suffer from this condition, which signifies a spike in blood sugar levels. Most moms-to-be with gestational diabetes go on to birth healthy children, but sugar levels must be monitored to prevent health problems in both Mom and Baby, and complications such as preterm birth. If you don't pass the first screening, you may need to do a three-hour glucose test. Bottoms up.

Red blood cell (RBC) or antibody screening: Your blood type and Rh factor may differ from your baby's. This test checks if this is the case, and if so, if you have developed antibodies to your baby's blood. If you have, you may be injected with Rh immune globulin to prevent those antibodies from attacking your baby.

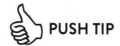 **PUSH TIP**

If you're opting for a hospital birth, this is a good time to register for admission.

35–37 Weeks

Group B strep (GBS) screening: This involves a swab of the vagina and rectum to check for GBS, a type of bacterial infection that occurs in about 25 percent of healthy pregnant women. Even though GBS is *not* a sexually transmitted disease, it can be passed on to Baby during delivery, posing a serious threat to him. The most common complications are sepsis, pneumonia, and meningitis. If you test positive, you may require IV antibiotics during delivery.

EDUCATION IS THE MOST POWERFUL WEAPON

For myriad reasons, many women choose to forgo various doctor's visits, ultrasounds, and/or tests. Now that you know what they are, you can delve a little deeper and make informed decisions about your body, your pregnancy, and your baby.

You have many more choices ahead of you—things like deciding on your fantasy delivery team, whether to circumcise, and even where to labor. Don't worry—we'll cover all of those in *Chapter 8: Labor a la Carta: Eeny, Meeny, Miny, Moe...Mi Mamá Picks the Very Best One.*

For now, let's just relish the wonderful news you've got to share: You're having a baby!

Disseminating the News

Once I was in the clear, I couldn't wait to tell the world I was finally going to be a mom. I wanted to tell my family in person, so I made plans to visit Puerto Rico over Thanksgiving to do that. I did break the rules by telling them on week 11—I couldn't really reschedule a national holiday.

My dad and I love to drink wine together. We went to the bar. In front of our female bartender, he asked me what I wanted. "Nothing," I told. "I'm pregnant." At which point, he could've downed a shot. The bartender was thrilled. In her entire career, she had never heard a girl tell her father she was pregnant, while on the job. But then again, not a lot of father/daughter relationships are fermented in good Spanish wine.

When I told my mom and youngest sister, we laughed, cried, and jumped up and down like in a cartoon. I then had to survive a weeklong cruise with them, crammed into the same little room together. My mom snores like a whale and I couldn't drink myself through the night. It was a long seven days.

The twelve-week mark fell right around Christmas, when we flew to Georgia visit my in-laws for the holidays. We again waited until they offered me a glass of wine to nonchalantly tell them that I shouldn't drink during my first trimester. My mother-in-law almost fell off her chair. She had been waiting for her first grandchild since before I had held my first Cabbage Patch.

I wish we would've planned out more creative ways to tell our families. But at the time, the pregnant news seemed enough of a surprise coming from us thirty-something "liberal L.A. people."

If you're into elaborate reveals, you could have a lot of fun coming out of the pregnancy closet. I've included ideas for you to draw from, which I'm also saving in case there's ever a baby number two.

WAYS TO SHARE THE PREGNANT NEWS

Here are some fun ways to "show" rather than tell. Some may fit your personality more than others, so select at will!

For the Social Media Butterflies:

- Post that positive test on your newsfeed. "Likes" & "Loves" guaranteed!

- If you have a pet, dress her up in a onesie, put a rattle in her mouth, and post with the caption: "Spot is already jealous."

- Write it in the sand and snap a pic for Instagram.

- Stage a photo of your partner passed out next to booze with the positive pregnancy test in hand.

- If you already have a child, post of photo of them in a "Big Sister" t-shirt or holding a sign saying "Big Brother in the Works." Or record a short video of them making the announcement—not only will you melt a lot of hearts, but it's a surefire way to include your older child in the journey.

- Get the reaction on camera. Take your partner/mom/best friend into a photo booth or prep them for a group shot and say "1...2...3...I'm pregnant!" and then snap it. Or surreptitiously shoot a video through the whole thing, then hashtag it and post it!

- Take a picture of yourself with a fake belly and post with the caption: "Me in nine months." Photoshop in a DeLorean, and it may go viral.

- Post a picture of a bun in the oven.

For the Retro Hipsters:

- Did you know you can still send a singing or hand-delivered paper telegram?!

- Deliver a message in a bottle to someone's front door.

- Whisper it in someone's ear. I find this to be such a simple, sweet, and intimate way to share the news.

For the Socially Unreserved:

- Tie a bunch of balloons to a relative's car announcing they are grandparents/aunt-and-uncle/whatever to-be.

- At a sporting event, ask them to announce it through the speaker system or feature you holding up a sign so you can have someone watching on the other end of the TV.

- Add your baby's ultrasound to your PowerPoint work presentation.

For the Pranksters:

- Get a recording of a baby crying and have it go off in the middle of the night. When your partner wakes up, you can simply say: "Get used to it."

- Have a surplus of diapers delivered to your partner's office or home. (Just make sure you're there when it arrives if you want to see the reaction!)

- Hide a message in a fortune cookie that reads: "I foresee a lot of shit in your future."

- Freeze a miniature plastic baby inside an ice cube and pour your partner a stiff drink over it. You can call it "Baby on the Rocks."

For the Puzzle-Solving Enthusiasts:

- Plan a scavenger hunt that leads the puzzle-solver to the baby section of a store; the playground; a remote spot with a staged fake stork; or to finding a bun in the oven.

- Put a stack of family movie classics in front of the TV: *Knocked Up, Look Who's Talking, Three Men and a Baby, Parenthood, Home Alone,* etc. (Don't include *Rosemary's Baby* or *The Hand That Rocks the Cradle* in the bunch unless you're into very dark humor.)

DIVULGE OR DELAY?

It's up to you when to share the pregnant news with friends and family. I'm an over-sharer, so keeping the secret was hard. And if I do this again, I don't know that I *would* withhold the information so long, especially around loved ones whose support I'd need if something went wrong.

Yet, a good reason to delay imparting the precious information is to avoid the barrage of unsolicited advice and commentary you'll receive: *You're not showing; are you sure there's a baby in there? (Yup. Pretty darn positive.) Your belly looks like it'll be a boy. (You don't say.) You can't wear stilettos. (Yes, I can, though not sure I want to.) Don't raise your hands over your head or the umbilical cord will get tangled up around your baby's neck. (Old Wives' Tales 101.) I don't think you wanna eat that sushi. (I do!) You shouldn't really be exercising. (Yes, I should—it's good for me and the baby.) You can't go to a rock concert. (Why the heck not?!)*

The list goes on and on. We'll delve into food advisories in *Chapter 3: Prenatal Health: Have Your Cake and Don't Eat It, Too.*

Praying for My Vagina and Soul

After I ran out of people to tell I was pregnant, the fear of pushing a baby out of my vagina and becoming a parent reared its head.

Is my preoccupation worse than the actual ring of fire? I wondered. *What about motherhood? Do I have what it takes?*

"Are you scared?" My husband asked one day, referring to childbirth.

I told him what I had been telling myself: "Not really—our bodies were meant to do this. Women have been giving birth for thousands of years."

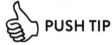 **PUSH TIP**

Do not Google everything that could go wrong with your pregnancy.

But in reality, I lay in bed night after night, sweating over my idealistic drug-free vaginal delivery. I pondered how giving birth stacked up next to passing meteoric shit matter while horribly constipated. If I could survive labor-long dumps that left me walking bow-legged with a bloody A-hole, I could survive childbirth, right? *RIGHT? Oh God, what if I rip from the front through to the back and end up with a vaganus? Please, God, don't let me get a fourth-degree tear. In the name of the Father, and of the Son, and of the Holy Spirit. Amen.*

If going through the pregnancy song and dance and then pushing out a baby was scary, the thought of becoming a mother was terrifying. Especially having told my husband that I was always meant to be a mom. I had set myself up for prominence.

WTF have I gotten myself into? I worried. Which is the title of the next chapter.

WTF HAVE I GOTTEN MYSELF INTO?

Birth Your Own "Mamafesto"

I'M NOT A PSYCHIC. I think horoscopes are silly fun and I tend to believe science over faith. But I just *knew* I would have a girl.

I felt genetically predisposed, you see. Like most women in my family, I have a tilted uterus. My mother had three girls, and her own mother had five. Female spermatozoa (plural form of sperm) tend to be slower and more cautious. They are more likely to traverse a tilted uterus and infiltrate a fertile egg. Lady sperm are marathoners. Male sperm tend to rush in and crash before the finish line—they're all about the sprint.

On October 6, 2013, a lonely spermatozoon loaded with my husband's DNA and gender-defining chromosomes went up slow and steady like a lonesome cowgirl and lassoed into my egg. A girl was indeed conceived the tried and true old-fashioned way.

But was I ready to raise her? Did I have the right stuff to do it well? Every day I carried her in my womb, I worried I would end up with a daughter like me: a runaway teen.

Benefits of the Doubt

I have always been lousy at following rules. Before age ten, I had cut a boy's cheek with scissors, gotten busted gluing crayon boxes together at the store, and almost lost a limb riding the handrail on an airport escalator. I was the girl who always got sent to the principal's office. By the time I was seventeen, I had gone to five different high schools and run away from home. (More on that in *Chapter 15: Dogged Mommy Guilt: Bite It Before It Bites You.*) I was horrible all the way up until I got my GED, months after all my peers had graduated from legit educational institutions, at which time I settled for just plain bad.

In my twenties, I managed to get my shit together, at least enough to become a mediocre, somewhat accountable adult. I finished college, survived grad school, traveled through Europe, lived in Asia, and then settled into a "real" job in the U.S. In my thirties, I married my husband, bought a house, and made a home. On paper, I was ready to have a child.

Problem was, for thirty-five years I had never been successfully responsible for another living organism—plant or pet. My husband was no better. He hadn't even held a baby in his entire life. We'd tried to get a dog together once, but had ended up adopting him out to a nice avocado-farming couple who, we realized, could give our mutt, Martin Scorsese, a much better life than we could.

We were a solid couple, but we still lived like college students, burning the work/party candle at both ends. I knew this would all change with parenthood, but how much?

What if I resent my baby for taking all that away from me? I agonized. *What does "all" mean? What if I end up hating being a mom?* This was not like all those other things in life I had signed up for and quit: dance, tennis, guitar, sailing, scuba diving, smoking, dog-owning, Catholicism. Of course, I had picked a hell of a time to second-guess my parental capacity. Timing has never been my forte.

The Birth of the Mamafesto

To avoid suffering a nervous breakdown, I had to sit myself down for a pep talk. I reminded myself what had gotten me here in the first place: love. I had loved my daughter before she was even conceived. That was a start, right? I then asked myself: What does it really mean—*to me*—to be a good parent?

Asking myself this question was key to helping me find my inner mama. It helped me focus on the big picture—life—and not on whether I was equipped to find the right preschool that would get my daughter into Harvard.

A rule-breaker at heart, I figured the only way I could follow some sort of guidelines would be if I wrote my own. So I sat down and drafted my own "Mamafesto": a set of guiding principles to remind me of what was important to *me* and help me navigate the tempestuous waters of motherhood.

MY MAMAFESTO

I, Ivette, your mom, promise...

○ *To love you unconditionally and infinitely. My love for you is like the universe: forever expanding. I will be very verbal about this. I apologize in advance for not curbing my affection in front of your friends.*

○ *To always look out for your well-being, health, and safety. But if we need oxygen on a plane, I'll have to attach my mask first in order to better help you. If you have a kid someday, I hope you will do the same—whether on a plane or in a more figurative way.*

○ *To make a conscious effort to be present every time I am around you.*

○ *To respect your feelings and consider your thoughts no matter how vehemently I disagree with them. Or how much they hurt me.*

○ *To cultivate your trust like the most sacred of gardens, because I want you to always walk knowing that I've got your back.*

○ *To believe IN you unfailingly, even when I don't believe you. I know you'll lie someday and even though I'm sure it'll sting, I will try to understand your reasons—if you're caught, that is. I don't intend for you to be a pro at lying, but I do hope that if you have to do it, you know how to do it well. Sometimes the truth is better left unsaid. Other times, it calls to be screamed at the top of your lungs.*

○ *To encourage you to listen to your gut. As you grow older, it will advise you. It will lead you where you want to go and hopefully steer you away from trouble. If I'm honest, my gut has led me down some pretty questionable roads, but other times I've gotten into trouble for not listening to it. Which brings me to my next promise.*

○ *To teach you (and me) not to fear your mistakes. And to help you keep your chin high after a fall. It's not our mistakes but how we fix and overcome them that makes us better than average.*

○ *To impart that being wise is knowing that you'll never know it all.*

○ *To push myself to do the hard thing when the easy option isn't the best for you.*

○ *To stimulate your imagination. "Only boring people get bored," my Abuelo used to say.*

○ *To encourage you to express yourself through art, whatever form may feel right to you.*

○ *To listen to you so we can educate each other.*

○ *To remind myself every time I want to bitch about someone that tolerance leads to freedom. So I can help you see the world without judgment. Maybe you can help me do that, too.*

○ *To guide you to be compassionate to friends and strangers, yet cautious, because unfortunately not everyone means well.*

○ *To never avoid apologizing to you and others. A sincere apology is as important as true forgiveness.*

○ *To show you the importance of being grateful for what we have and for what we don't.*

○ *To teach you to fight fairly. Some things are worth the brawl.*

○ *To impress upon you the significance of keeping your feet on the ground and your head in the clouds, so you can steadily march on towards your wildest dreams.*

○ *To make you aware that there will always be something that will slip through your fingers, but that the gained experience is usually worth the loss.*

○ *To train you to fold fitted sheets neatly so that you can impress your future love.*

○ *To encourage you to appreciate sarcasm and arm you with humor, even when deemed inappropriate. A family that laughs together...*

○ *To do everything in my power for you to experience more love, health, and happiness than I've ever had.*

○ *To be an example of someone who is not defined or limited by gender, sexual orientation, race, ethnicity, or social status. Just by the humanity we all share.*

○ *To help you grow up to be the person you want to be.*

○ *To see the world through your eyes every chance I get, but to hold back when you need to see it alone.*

Reading my Mamafesto over and over helps me to stay focused on what's important, forgive myself when I mess up, and continue forging—and enjoying—my own motherhood adventure.

WRITE YOUR OWN MAMAFESTO

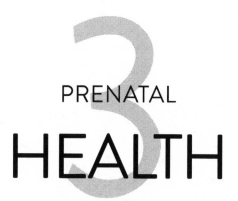

PRENATAL
HEALTH

Have Your Cake and Don't Eat It, Too

S OME FRIENDS MAY SAY: "You're not fat—you're pregnant!" Those words may be true, and they can bring great comfort during times of pregnant-body-image angst. So I hate to be a Debbie Downer on the matter, but...these are not mutually exclusive conditions.

We can be fat *and* pregnant.

Contrary to popular belief, being pregnant does not come with a free license to eat everything on the menu. This is terribly tempting, but unhealthy for both Mom and Baby.

The Centers for Disease Control and Prevention (CDC) Maternal and Infant Health Branch recently cited that nearly 50 percent of women gain more than the recommended 35 pounds during pregnancy. If you're already overweight, your doctor may even recommend gaining only 11 to 25. Exceeding these standards could complicate your pregnancy and after-birth, and make it really hard for you to return to your normal weight afterwards (no matter what you hear about breastfeeding!).

That said, it's most important to focus on your health and the size of the baby during pregnancy, not on the number glaring back at you on the scale. Tell that scale that you're the one pushing!

Average Pregnancy Weight Gain

5–9 lbs.   Pure baby (by end of pregnancy)

1–2 lbs.   Yummy placenta

2 lbs.   Uterus (it grows like a Chia Pet)

2 lbs.   Boobage

4 lbs.   Blood

2 lbs.   Amniotic fluid

5–7 lbs.   Storage in Mom's cells
(fats, nutrients, and protein)

3–4 lbs.   Other bodily fluids

Perpetuating the Lie

I'm a slob. I don't bother with my hair, I don't file or paint my nails, and makeup overwhelms me. As a result, my nails look like brittle flying saucers (short, rectangular, with clingy cuticles that I neglect). My hair is usually smattered with gray strays and at least one unintentional dread, as I never brush it (hardly ever wash it, either). Most of my clothes have been gifted or handed down to me by the people who know it's the only way I'll wear new outfits. Everything else is vintage—and not in the cool way, but because I've actually had them since the nineties. And this morning, I threw on the stained jeans from the floor that make my butt look saggy over the shirt I slept in (that I also happened to wear all day yesterday), slipped my unmanicured toes into a pair of flip-flops, and went to the bank. I didn't even wash my face.

I'm telling you all of this so you can perhaps forgive me when you read the following sentence: I gained only nineteen pounds during my pregnancy and was back into my old jeans just two weeks after giving birth to my very healthy eight-pound, six-ounce baby.

Cry me a river, I know.

But before you punch me, know that I don't have a personal trainer, a private chef, or some magic Hollywood diet pills. But I did carve out the time to exercise and commit to eating healthy throughout my pregnancy. *Am I insane?* Maybe. But I feel my best when I am strong and fit. I wasn't going to let my pregnancy change that, and I was amazed at the results that a little discipline elicited— well, actually, a *lot* of discipline.

However, for a while, I dismissed compliments (and good-natured disgruntlement) about my post-baby figure, claiming apologetically: "I just got lucky." But then I realized that with that big, fat LIE, I was perpetuating the notion that fitness just "happens" to some people. I couldn't continue giving fate and biology that much credit when the truth was I had worked my butt off before, during, and after my pregnancy to stay in shape.

I'm not one of those infuriating women who eats heart-attack-inducing double cheeseburgers and supersize fries, exercises poolside with mimosas, drinks milkshakes for dinner, and looks bored when saying: "I just have a fast metabolism." *Those* girls need to be spanked, either for abusing the bodies they've been blessed with or for lying about where they put everything they eat. If the latter, they need to be force-fed bacon until they're about to burst so we can make pâté out of their bulimic asses.

I can say this because I used to be one of them.

Never Say Die-t

I used to be fat. Kids chanted a custom-written Miss Piggy song just for me, sung to the beat of *Ghostbusters*. To get away from them, I spent a lot of time in Nurse Belky's infirmary room pretending to be sick.

Thanks to these bullies and my low self-esteem, I battled an eating disorder throughout most of my teens and into my twenties. So, yeah, my diligence and passion for fitness is deeply rooted in some fucked-up issues. But the only way I was able to get myself "clean" was to change my relationship with food and to make exercise an enjoyable part of my life. After surviving many canned-beet diet fads in the nineties and struggling with bulimia for ten years, I've finally found a semi-healthy lifestyle that works for me. This includes indulging in decadent salads, too much wine, and daily nibbles of dark chocolate. I eat well and exercise (a lot), but I'm not a boot-camp rat, I don't skimp too much on carbs, and I never, ever use the word diet.

Diets are not suitable for former bulimics or pregnant women. I know of a pregnant girl who ate salads without dressing for almost every meal. That just takes pregnancy to a new level of misery. You NEED to eat. A starved mom = an unhealthy child. Good food is necessary for your baby's brain, especially during the first half of your pregnancy.

With the exception of doctor-recommended nutritional guidelines and/or restrictions, *a pregnant woman never diets*. Here are some compelling reasons why:

- Poor nutrition during pregnancy can cause abnormalities in your baby's endocrine functioning and organ development, and can stunt your baby's metabolism.

- Some toxins are stored in fat cells, away from your vital organs. When you lose weight, these toxins are released from your fat stores into your blood, where they can move across the placenta and reach your fetus.

- You'll be hungry all the time. Why on earth would you want to diet?

The proof is not in the pudding, ladies—it's in the serving size.

Size Matters

Throughout pregnancy, we moms-to-be hear variations of "now you have to eat for two." This is *not* true. So be ready to educate your once-removed second cousin Zelda when she tells you to help yourself to another serving of mac 'n' cheese because she:

a. is misinformed.

b. likes to repeat shit she heard from other folk who heard from other folk.

c. wants to eat vicariously through you.

d. secretly enjoys seeing other people gain weight.

e. all of the above.

You can explain to Zelda that at worst (and Vagina Fairy conspiring) your baby might be fourteen pounds full-term. (But take solace that most babies average only seven and a half pounds.) Does that really qualify as a full-sized human you need to nourish? Most experts recommend that during the second trimester of carrying a single baby, you consume approximately 300 calories per day over your standard daily allotment. Double that if you're pregnant with twins. During your third trimester, you may increase your caloric intake by 500 a day for each baby in your belly.

While pregnant, I got away with consuming a hearty 2,500–3,000 calories a day because I remained active and ate healthy foods. The quantity of calories and fats we eat are not as important as their source. For example, an avocado may have the same caloric content as a Häagen-Dazs Vanilla & Almond Bar. And, in fact, the avocado has more fat than the ice cream! However, the ice cream bar has 13 grams of saturated fats (65 percent the recommended daily intake) and 19 grams of sugar—almost 100 percent of the suggested daily allowance. On the other hand, the fats in the avocado are mainly monosaturated (the best kind) and the sugar content is about half a gram. Not to mention that avocados are jam-packed with fiber and important nutrients (folate, potassium, vitamin E, and magnesium). So if you throw an avocado into one side of the health ring and the Häagen-Dazs ice cream bar into the other...who wins? Avocado knocks out Häagen-Dazs's melted sat-fat ass in round one!

Fat gets blamed for all sorts of evil, but not all fats are created equal. Good fats are vital for nutrient absorption, and help the placenta and other tissues grow. They help nourish a fetus's developing brain and eyes, and build his immune system. It's important to consume good fats while pregnant. Check out this glossary of fats:

THE SKINNY ON FATS

saturated

It is recommended to avoid these because they increase the levels of bad cholesterol (LDL) in your blood. However, because I didn't have any cholesterol issues, I indulged in natural sources of saturated fat while pregnant.

"Sat fats" are found in many animal-based foods such as red meat, poultry, lard, butter, cheese, whole milk, whole milk products, and in palm and palm kernel oil, coconut oil, cocoa butter, and the infamous partially hydrogenated oils.

During and after my pregnancy, I made sure to eat quality foods rich in saturated fats (something frowned upon in some low-fat-advocating circles). If you're not vegan, antibiotic-free dairy and meat products provide good sources of protein, iron, zinc, and B vitamins, and are part of a balanced diet when consumed with vegetables and whole grains.

When I craved red meat, I ate it. And I craved it a lot. Also, I'm a bit of a mouse when it comes to cheese; I probably ate an entire wheel in nine months. However, I didn't go full-fat on the milk and avoided partially hydrogenated oils altogether...except when I craved those damned Fig Newtons they sold in my office building.

polyunsaturated

"Poly fats" are considered good fats. They lower your body's cholesterol and are often loaded with vitamin E along with omega-6 and omega-3—fatty acids that your pregnant body needs, but can't produce. For optimal health, omega-3s should be consumed in higher quantities than omega-6s.

Poly fats are found mainly in fatty fish such as salmon, but also in corn, sesame, cottonseed, safflower, soybean, flaxseed, certain nuts, and sunflower oils.

Note: Be mindful of poly fats if you have low cholesterol. They can be tricky, as they reduce both bad and good cholesterol (HDL).

monosaturated

"Mono fats" are the alpha fats, so go nuts (*and* eat nuts!) while you're pregnant. Your baby's brain will thrive on mono fats. You can binge on olive oil (best when not heated), avocados, olives, nuts, nut oils, and nut butters. But hold back on the jelly: Sugar is Frenemy #1.

trans fat

Frenemy #2. Trans fats are produced when hydrogen is added to oil to solidify it (hydrogenation). Why are trans fats bad? The short scientific explanation is that the process of hydrogenation leads to the oil acting like a saturated fat, thus raising the blood cholesterol levels (i.e., LDL increases while HDL decreases). As mentioned, some sat fats aren't so terrible if you don't have cholesterol issues and, granted, small doses of trans fats appear naturally in some foods. However, trans fat are usually found in food with little to no nutritional value: margarines, shortenings, prepackaged cookies, frostings, pies, pastries, doughnuts, and fried foods. If you're a child of the nineties, when fluorescent fat-free cheddar pretzels populated the supermarket aisles, you probably ingested enough trans fats to last a lifetime. I know I did.

You CAN'T Eat...but I ate some of it anyway

This book has the word "renegade" in its title because I'm not prone to following directions and dislike being told I'm not allowed to do something. Thankfully, I have a considerably open-minded doctor who supported my decision to eat sushi and deli meats throughout my pregnancy. Preparation and safe-handling are the most important factors to heed when considering eating items on the "prohibited" list. But if consuming any of these foods makes you—or your doctor—the teeniest bit uncomfortable, wait 'til you pop that baby out to indulge.

Cold cuts. If you heat up the meat in a pan or the oven, you'll kill any chance of listeria, which makes it safe. My doc also claims that if you get fresh cuts at a reputable deli and eat them right away, you should be fine.

Unpasteurized cheese, juice, or milk. A small risk of listeria also lurks in unpasteurized dairy and beverages. As with cold cuts, you can melt your cheese to eliminate risk of listeriosis. I went French and disregarded this advice, *for cheese only*. I spread it nice and cold on a baguette. Not that you should, but I've lived to tell the story.

Raw eggs. For risk of salmonella. Good-bye, Caesar salad (though not all Caesar dressings are actually made with unpasteurized eggs). However, overcooked eggs aren't as optimal for your health because you kill all the good stuff, so I like to prepare mine a little runny, or even poached from time to time.

Also, be aware that bacteria lurks in the shell of a raw egg, so safe-handling practices include washing your egg and dropping it in a bowl of water before cracking it. If air bubbles emerge from the shell, the egg may have been compromised and that egg's better eaten well done or not at all.

You CAN Eat...and I ate most of these

Sushi. Again, safe handling is key, so find a trusted outlet. And stick to fish low in mercury. More on this ahead!

Smoked salmon. U.K. guidelines deem canned or shelf-safe smoked salmon okay to eat while pregnant.

Hot dogs and other cured meats. If you want to be extra healthy about it, limit your intake and look for high-quality dogs. Just not at the ballpark.

Coffee. Yes, you *can* eat—er, drink—it. (Though chomping on chocolate-covered coffee beans is amazing, too.) Experts recommend no more than twelve ounces of caffeine a day, which is a large-size cup of joe.

Plating Up

Consuming nutrient-rich food is even more important than avoiding empty calories—especially for your baby's brain. So I've compiled a list of important nutrients to consume while pregnant. Consult an expert to help you select the best nutrition plan and prenatal vitamins for you.

FOLATE OR FOLIC ACID

Folic acid shouldn't be confused with folate. Folate is the pure form of this vitamin found in food sources. Folic acid is the synthetic version that is found in most supplements.

Folic acid won't always convert into usable forms of folate, and it may not seep into the placenta like the real deal. That said, folic acid is better than no folate at all. Folic acid is good. Folate is better.

Why do I need it?

Folate is the most essential vitamin to consume while pregnant. This water-soluble, B-complex vitamin is essential for cell division and healthy red blood cells. It is the maestro orchestrating the DNA, making new, beautiful, smart baby cells. In fact, start taking this vitamin the instant you decide you want to get pregnant, as it may help you conceive faster.

Studies have found a correlation between low levels of folate and neural tube defects such as spina bifida, a congenital condition in which part of the spinal cord and its meninges are exposed through a gap in the backbone that could lead to various mental handicaps.

Low levels of folate may also cause miscarriage, paralysis of the lower limbs, anencephaly (when parts of the brain and skull are missing), premature birth, and low birthweight. Studies also indicate that taking folic acid may help prevent cleft lip and palate.

How much do I need?

The recommended dietary allowance (RDA) for folic acid or folate during pregnancy is 400–600 micrograms (mcg)/day. The max is 1,000 mcg. Don't exceed this recommendation. Too much folate or folic acid could cover up a B12 deficiency, which is associated with infertility and miscarriage.

Where can I find it?

Find folate in lemons, bananas, strawberries, avocados, romaine lettuce, dried beans, lentils, quinoa, peas, asparagus, okra, citrus fruits, papaya, fortified cereals, and dark green vegetables such as spinach, collard greens, brussels sprouts, broccoli, and turnip greens.

Most prenatals do come with the recommended dose of folate or folic acid, so there should be no need to take an extra pill.

OMEGA-3 / DHA

Omega-3s are essential fatty acids that appear to be key contributors to cognitive and behavioral functions. DHA (short for docosahexaenoic acid) is the omega-3 responsible for visual and neurological development. Our body doesn't produce omega-3s, so it is important to make sure we take in enough.

Why do I need it?

Babies that don't get enough DHA/omega-3s may develop vision and nerve problems.

How much do I need?

The International Society for the Study of Fatty Acids and Lipids (ISSFAL) recommends a minimum of 300 mg/day for pregnant and lactating women.

Where can I find it?

Fish is the biggest source of omega-3. While some fish are high in mercury and should be avoided, there are still plenty of fish in the sea that are safe to consume. This includes wild salmon, shrimp, sardines, tilapia, scallops, oysters, and squid. Vegan sources of omega-3 are algae, krill, avocados, chia seeds, and nut oils.

BIG NO-NO!

What's the Dealio with Mercurio?

Mercury may damage your baby's brain and nervous system, especially in the womb.

Fish with high levels of mercury include swordfish, shark, king mackerel, tilefish, marlin, orange roughy, and ahi tuna.

Most prenatals don't contain sufficient, or any, DHA. Seek an additional high-quality supplement to ensure you're getting the recommended daily allowance. Poor quality fish oils may be highly processed and contain heavy metals, PCBs, and dioxins. The good stuff is usually amber-colored and is lab-certified for purity. I love the brand, New Chapter for all things vitamins, and their DHA is made with extra-virgin wild Alaskan salmon oil. I've also taken Nordic Naturals and Rainbow Light Nutritional Systems—both reputable brands, as well.

PROTEIN

Proteins are an essential part of any living organism. They are structural components of body tissues such as muscle, hair, and collagen, composed of one or more long chains of amino acids. Amino acids are the building blocks of our human bodies—they handle most critical cell functions such as repairing muscle tissue and red blood cells, by serving as our internal Über, transporting nutrients and oxygen to and from cells.

Why do I need it?

Protein is vital to the health of your baby and may reduce the risk of birth defects. Furthermore, it plays a big role in Baby's hair and fingernail growth. Proteins are also believed to help Mom control blood-clotting around the uterus and placenta, and aid her body in producing iron.

How much do I need?

The APA recommends women consume 75 to 100 grams of protein a day while pregnant. Doctors may recommend that you up this if you have a high-risk pregnancy.

Eating enough good protein was important to me, so I upped my protein intake during pregnancy, though I didn't really adhere to a number.

Where can I find it?

Protein is mainly associated with animal products and by-products.

Soy and quinoa may be the only non-animal sources that pack all nine essential amino acids. Other seeds (quinoa is a seed) and grains also pack sufficient amounts of protein, including amaranth, spelt, teff, kamut, and sorghum. Soy-made products such as tempeh, tofu, and milk can also fulfill your protein quota.

A recovering vegetarian, I'm still a big fan of nuts and beans. In fact, while in grad school, my now-husband nicknamed me "Beans." Some of my classmates even wrote a song entitled "Beans García," which was much more endearing than the Miss Piggy ditty that plagued me in middle school. And for the record, my nickname was *not* bestowed upon me for any gassy incidents (I kept those private, pre-pregnancy), but simply for my love of the food that makes you toot.

If you're averse to eating natural protein sources and want to up your intake, you can turn to protein-supplemented shakes. However, pregnant and breastfeeding women should stay away from whey protein unless recommended by a doctor, due to lack of evidence about its long-term safety. Also steer clear of protein drinks designed for athletes, since they may contain herbs that are not compatible with pregnancy or breastfeeding. Protein powders specifically geared for pregnant and breastfeeding moms are available in the market, or you can always make your own protein-packed shake at home. My vegetarian friend makes a delicious one with plain yogurt, cocoa powder, raw almond butter, and banana.

Another trick to boost protein intake is to add white navy beans to your smoothie. They add a creamy texture but don't change the flavor. One cup contains 15 grams of protein.

CALCIUM WITH MAGNESIUM OR VITAMIN D

Your baby will steal calcium from your bones if you don't ingest enough, and rightfully so! They need it to grow strong bones and teeth, and a healthy ticker, nerves, and muscles. But Mama needs it too, so you do need to take calcium for two while pregnant.

Most nutrients need help being absorbed, and that's why it is essential to take calcium with magnesium or vitamin D.

Magnesium may help with bowel movements, which may be a perk, because for some of us pregnancy slows things down. However, I found that some magnesium blends gave me gas. Beans García in *da* house!

Why do I need it?

As aforementioned, if your baby doesn't have enough calcium, she will take it from your bones, putting you at risk for osteoporosis. Furthermore, a study cited by the World Health Organization (WHO) concluded that calcium supplementation more than halved the risk of preeclampsia.

How much do I need?

For pregnant and lactating women over age nineteen, the RDA for calcium is 1,000 mg/day (it's 1,300 if you're 14–18). For magnesium, the RDA is 400 mg for pregnant women ages 14–19, 350 mg ages 19–30, and 360 mg if you're 31–50 years of age.

Where can I find it?

You can boost your intake with calcium-and-vitamin D-fortified OJ, cow's milk (though the body absorbs non-dairy sources of calcium better), almond milk, rice milk, soy milk, coconut milk, bok choy, broccoli, broccoli rabe, collard greens, cucumbers, kale, okra, turnip greens, collard greens, spinach, romaine lettuce, edamame, tofu, sea vegetables, sardines (truly slimy but a superfood), salmon, figs, oranges, white beans, almonds, and sesame seeds.

Most prenatals don't have the recommended dose of calcium. So, yeah, you may need to invest in yet another tub of vitamins. Read the label to make sure it says calcium carbonate—the easiest kind for your body to absorb—and make sure it's lead-free. I like the Rainbow Light Nutritional Systems Calcium with Magnesium & Vitamin D3, though at 500 mg per tablet, it doesn't add up to the recommended 1,000 mg unless you double up, which would then make you exceed the recommendation for magnesium (since each tablet contains 250 mg). So I made sure to eat enough calcium-rich foods to supplement my supplements!

IRON

Your pregnant body needs extra iron to make enough hemoglobin for you and your baby. Hemoglobin is the red blood cell protein that shuttles oxygen into your organs and tissues. You need to consume enough iron to support the healthy growth of your baking bun.

Why do I need it?

It is estimated that half of all women suffer from anemia, an iron deficiency, during pregnancy. Anemia has been associated with preterm labor and low birthweight.

Iron also helps your body displace lead, a neurotoxin. Lead exposure has been linked to decreased IQ levels in children.

How much do I need?

It's recommended that you consume 27–44 mg of iron per day. Higher doses may cause digestive side effects such as nausea and vomiting—something a pregnant lady doesn't need! Furthermore, iron can be toxic in high levels, so never exceed the recommended amount.

Where can I find it?

The most easily absorbed iron, heme iron, is found in red meat, fish, poultry, and oysters. Therefore, if you are vegan or vegetarian, iron is a particularly important supplement to take.

Non-heme iron, which is harder to absorb, lives in iron-fortified cereal, oatmeal, pumpkin seeds, molasses, spirulina, spinach, raisins, lentils, chickpeas, navy beans, black beans, kindey beans, edamame, and tofu.

If you combine heme and hon-heme, you'll absorb a good percentage of iron. So bring on the beef chili!!! Additionally, cooking in a cast iron pan will add a significant amount of the compound to your food.

To help your body soak up iron, you can scarf down some vitamin C (found in bell peppers, hot peppers, thyme, parsley, and leafy greens). Calcium, on the other hand, makes it harder for your body to absorb iron, especially if you're iron-deficient.

Most prenatals have enough iron for pregnant women but not enough calcium. This is fine, because it's best you take them separately anyway. Take a calcium supplement at least two hours before or after your prenatal to ensure your body is absorbing enough of each mineral.

VITAMIN D

Vitamin D is what your body makes when exposed to sunlight. Recent studies indicate that you can even absorb vitamin D while wearing SPF 15 sunscreen. However, our lifestyles don't always allow us the luxury to step outside two to three times a week, and some of us still fear sunburn. If this is the case, we may need supplements.

Why do I need it?

Vitamin D's main role is to keep calcium and phosphorous levels up to standard. Some researchers believe that a vitamin D deficiency could hinder your baby's bone development, causing growth retardation and skeletal deformities, and could reduce your child's immune function through adulthood. A shortage of vitamin D during pregnancy has also been linked to a greater risk of preeclampsia for Mom.

Vitamin D is now being studied widely for its preventative potential. It is believed to stave off type 1 diabetes, multiple sclerosis, rheumatoid arthritis, osteoarthritis, some cancers, gum disease, and high blood pressure. It may also ward off depression.

How much do I need?

Pregnant women need at least 600 IU ("International Units," a measure often used for vitamins) and up to 4,000 IU per day, according to the Vitamin D Council. New research suggests leaning towards the higher end of this range, as it may prevent preterm birth and infections.

Where can I find it?

For us carnivores, vitamin D lives in cod-liver oil and fatty fish such as catfish, salmon, mackerel, and sardines. Consumable vegetarian sources of vitamin D are yogurts, milk, eggs, and cheeses; vegan sources are orange juice and fortified cereals.

As far as supplements, vegetarians and vegans beware: Most vitamin D pills are sourced from lanolin, the grease found in lamb's wool. I love Natural Health Goodies Vitamin D3 Drops with MCT. MCT stands for medium-chain triglycerides, a synthetic substance that emulates the fatty acids found in coconut oil, which are believed to have many benefits, including helping restore metabolic function. For the record: Yes, I do think cold-pressed virgin coconut oil is great, but no, I don't think the fountain of youth gushed coconut oil—cold-pressed or not.

B6

Vitamin B6 synthesizes serotonin and norepinephrine to reduce stress, and helps form myelin, a protective layer that insulates the nerves.

Why do I need it?

Vitamin B6 works with folate and B12 in preventing neural tube defects in your baby, such as spina bifida and anencephaly. If, like me, you were on the pill for many years before trying to conceive, it's especially important to replenish your body's supply of this vitamin, as oral contraceptives may have depleted it. It is believed that vitamin B6 also helps fight morning sickness, but consult a physician before upping the recommended dosage.

How much do I need?

For pregnant women, the recommended daily allowance of vitamin B6 is 1.9 mg, but the maximum (for all adults) is as high as 100 mg. For breastfeeding mamas, the RDA goes up to 2 full mgs.

Where can I find it?

Foods like tuna, salmon, turkey breast, chicken, chickpeas, spinach, broccoli, onion, hazelnuts, raisins, winter squash, bulgur, asparagus, and bananas are rich in vitamin B6.

Most prenatal vitamins have sufficient B6, but double-check to make sure you're covered!

B12

Vitamin B12 is necessary for proper red blood cell formation, neurological function, and DNA synthesis. This vitamin crosses the placenta during pregnancy and is present in breast milk.

Why do I need it?

Some experts believe that a B12 deficiency can be as serious as an iron or folate deficiency. Undetected and untreated vitamin B12 deficiency in babies can result in neurological abnormalities. Low B12 has also been associated with preeclampsia and postnatal depression.

How much do I need?

The daily recommendation for pregnant women is 2.6 mcg. It goes up to 2.8 mcg for lactating moms.

Where can I find it?

Healthy doses of B12 are found in clams, trout, sockeye salmon, haddock, beef, beef liver, ham, chicken breast, eggs, milk, cheese, yogurt, and some fortified cereals.

B12 is generally absent in plant foods, so vegans need to take a supplement. For optimal absorption, choose one made of methylcobalamin and administered in spray form.

Supplementing the Cause

As alluded to above, besides practicing well-balanced nutrition, you may want to take supplemental vitamins. If so, make sure you're following the recommended dosage and familiarize yourself with the tolerable upper intake level (UL) of each. It is possible to overdose on certain vitamins and minerals, which could cause harm to you and your baby.

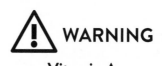 **WARNING**

Vitamin A

Even though vitamin A is necessary for your developing baby's lung, eye, and skin cell production, taking too much can be detrimental to his health. Exceeding 5,000 UI of vitamin A per day while pregnant may cause congenital birth defects. During breastfeeding, you can nearly double that.

When choosing dietary vitamin A or supplements, seek it in the form of mixed carotenoids rather than retinoids (animal sources), as retinoids build up in your body and can become toxic.

Natural carotenoid sources include butternut squash, cantaloupe, carrots, kale, mangoes, pumpkins, spinach, and sweet potatoes.

If you can, cough up the money to purchase food-based vitamins to ensure your body absorbs the maximum amount of nutrients. I swear by New Chapter's Perfect Prenatal Multivitamin, a whole-food probiotic culture supplement made with vegetables and herbs, which can be taken on an empty stomach. I know it hurts to spend ninety bucks on a tub of pills, but it may save you on medical bills later down the line. If you're nausea-ridden, chewable vitamin tablets may be your best bet.

Read On!

If you're into nutrition, I recommend reading:

Super Foods Rx For Pregnancy: The Right Choices for a Healthy, Smart, Super Baby by Steven Pratt, M.D.

This comprehensive nutritional guide is the first thing I hand out when someone tells me they're thinking of getting pregnant.

The Better Baby Book: How to Have a Healthier, Smarter, Happier Baby by Lana and David Asprey

Though the authors don't share my love for dairy; are way more hard-core about sugar and carbs than I am (coconut milk–sweetened rice seems to be the only treat Lana indulged in while pregnant); and cite some findings that are highly controversial, I garnered a lot of great nutritional tips from this book, such as putting a teaspoon of coconut oil into my morning brew.

Moderation Is Good...in Moderation

My definition of healthy is: pretty healthy. I try to be healthy at least 92 percent of the time. The other 8 percent, I'm either on vacation or eating as though I am.

When I found it too hard to be healthful during my pregnancy, I gave myself permission to indulge without guilt. During a business trip, I allowed myself a few chocolate-covered Oreos in a hotel bed to keep me sane while all my non-pregnant colleagues were partying at the hotel bar. After I was done (and had salvaged all the crumbs off the bedspread), I wanted to go downstairs and get more junk food—because that's what sugar does to one's brain—but I listened to the skinny angel on my shoulder (she looks like Bethenny Frankel) and popped a wad of gum instead and did butt-clenches while watching *Scandal*. Go NEAT! (See chart in next chapter.)

It was tough not to keep indulging, but I had to ask myself if I really needed to gorge on 2,080 empty calories while I watched Kerry Washington pretend she was gonna drink a goblet of wine and eat an entire bag of popcorn. The craving to binge was gone before the commercial break.

Traveling makes dietary decisions like this challenging because you're typically not surrounded by nutritious choices. If I'd been at home, I would've mixed plain 2-percent yogurt with nuts, lime zest, a little granola, and a nice helping of shredded coconut or raw honey. This would've satisfied my sweet tooth plus given me good fats, protein, fiber, and calcium.

While pregnant, I did snack a lot. I mirrored Olivia Pope and ate a ton of popcorn. I added parmesan cheese and white truffle oil to it. Sometimes I even paired it with a Polly Pocket–size glass of wine—just to give it that Olivia feel. I also indulged in red peppers or blue corn chips dipped in humus or guacamole, and apple slices with peanut butter. Trust me: It's not like I was eating celery sticks and raw broccoli while I was pregnant. I don't even eat that when I'm *not* pregnant.

Build-A-Snack

Mix 'n' match from the following to create your own
300–500-calorie snack:

Vegetables:

  Mushrooms, 1 cup (15)

  Raw spinach, 2 cups (14)

  Red bell pepper, 1/2 cup (30)

  Celery, 1 cup (16)

Fruit:

  Small banana (89)

  Small apple (80)

  Avocado, half (161)

  Strawberries, 1 cup (46)

Protein:

  Hard-boiled egg (78)

  Scrambled eggs, 2 (197)

  Sliced turkey breast, 2 oz. (50)

  Hummus, 2 Tbsp. (70)

  Peanut butter, 1 Tbsp. (95)

  Raw almonds, 1 oz. (164)

Dairy:

  Small plain fat-free Greek yogurt (100)

  Chocolate milk, 1 cup (158)

  Single cheese slice (70)

  Grated Parmesan cheese, 1 Tbsp. (22)

Carbohydrates:

  Granola, 1/3 cup (160)

  Pretzels, 1 oz. (110)

  Ak-mak 100% Whole Wheat Stone Ground Sesame Crackers, 5 (115)

Wheat bread, 1 slice (75)

Pita round, half large (190)

Air-popped popcorn, 1 cup, no butter (35)

Condiments:

Whole-grain mustard, 1 Tbsp. (10)

Mayonnaise, 1 Tbsp. (90)

Whipped topping,* 1 Tbsp. (11)

*I like Tru Whip, because it's a very "clean" brand of imitation whipped cream.

Olive oil, 1 Tbsp.* (120)

*Though I wouldn't worry too much about "overdosing" on OO.

Special Treats for Special Occasions:

Chips Ahoy cookie, 2 (96)

Fig Newton, 2 (110)

Ben & Jerry's Cherry Garcia Frozen Yogurt, 1/2 cup (200)

Häagen-Dazs Vanilla Ice Cream, 1/2 cup (270)

Vanilla milkshake, 1/2 small (265)

Kettle-cooked potato chips, 2 oz (300)

The Road to Wellville

Weight gain aside, your knocked-up body (breast tissue, hips, lower back, stomach skin, wrist, neck, vagina, nipples, brain, etc.) will be deconstructed during pregnancy, labor, breastfeeding, and motherhood in general. Your zygote will grow into a life-size baby in your womb, crushing all your organs and stretching your skin beyond Hannibal Lector's wildest dreams. And then, you'll get to push her out of your V-hole or get your skin and abdominal muscles sliced in order to release the alien that has been squatting in your uterus. (More wank-bank for Lector.) Then, she may destroy your already blackened and swollen nipples, give you carpal tunnel, and ruin all your dreams of beauty sleep.

Your body will never be what it was, so make peace with that as soon as you can; but know that you have the power to keep a healthy body and mind throughout your pregnancy.

Now, after you have your little one, maintaining control over your wellness may be more difficult. It's hard to find motivation to eat healthy after baby. Lack of sleep, postpartum blues, anxiety, boredom, or just all the casseroles your awesome friends and family have dropped off are all compelling reasons to eat irresponsibly. And if you're breastfeeding, you may be ravenous twenty-four hours a day. I've commiserated with many new "mombies" about eating sandwiches in the middle of the night after nursing our babies.

Eat when you're hungry. Choose nutritious and delicious food. Treat your body right. Your body just did the most amazing thing: It grew and brought a child into this world.

Like our babies, our bodies deserve kindness, patience, and understanding. You get to choose when to pull over at a rest stop, take a scenic detour, or push down on that pedal. Just understand that it may take a while to fit back into your jeans. In fact, one of my skinniest friends never did: Her hips stayed at "childbearing" width, and she now looks even better than she did prior to having kids!

When you eat well, you feel great. Combine that with the pregnancy "glow," and you're one hot pregnant mama.

It's also amazing what a little exercise can add to the equation. Which brings us to our next topic.

BRING IT ON, JANE FONDA

4

Keeping Your Pregnant Ass Fit
While Your Belly Gets Big

I'M SO OLD that I remember flipping through *Jane Fonda's Workout Book* to follow her routine in pictures. Now that technology makes exercise options even more accessible, there are few legit excuses not to work out while pregnant. Legit excuses include doctor's orders, crippling nausea, lower-back pain, and colossal hemorrhoids. Barring any such malady, your pregnancy is not an excuse to sit around on your ass all day. 'Tis not the season.

According to the American College of Obstetricians and Gynecologists, women can safely exercise for thirty minutes a day while pregnant. According to me, exercise involves sweat, a semi-challenging level of resistance, and clenched butt cheeks. However, I'm not a doctor, so please make sure to talk to yours first. Mine said I could continue any activity I was used to doing before becoming pregnant. And like a good patient, I followed his orders.

Did I wake up every morning like the Energizer Bunny, banging on my symbols, ready to hit the gym? Fuck no. I forced my pregnant ass into gear because it was important to me to keep my shared body healthy and in shape. I was able to exercise almost every day for the first 210 days of my 288-day pregnancy. This was mainly because collapsing on the couch was not as enticing without wine. The hardest thing about my pregnancy was laying off the booze for nine months. Also, I suffered almost no pregnancy side effects, like backaches, nausea, sleeping problems, swollen limbs, or severe leg cramps. I know—slap me. I was a lucky MF.

But if it's any consolation, I did run out of luck towards the end of my nine months, when I suffered the worst hemorrhoid outbreak ever known to my anus (and my A-hole has been around the H-block since it was sweet sixteen). In other words, I got beat.

Getting Beat

Let me introduce you to our family's "got beat" theory. Getting beat is winning the lottery of misfortune. It's when you are the subject of a cosmic injustice. These cruelties can't be blamed on karma, because at least then, you would deserve such a fate. Getting beat is when bad shit just randomly happens to you, through no fault of your own. For example, if you miss a connecting flight and get stuck at the airport with your toddler and then your iPad breaks: you got beat.

> "My poor vagina is so fat it shocks me. I looked down there with a mirror last night and was taken aback by how bad my hemorrhoids were, as well as how swollen my vulva and labia are, complete with big puffy varicose veins. It's a real horror show."
>
> —A.M., Film Editor, Los Angeles, CA,
> Pregnant with #2

About a week before my due date, parts of my butthole peeked outside of their bat cave. One of them was swollen to the size of a baby testicle. I couldn't walk, stand, or sit. I laid sideways and exercised my fingers on the remote control. Same fingers I was using to insert bullet-size suppositories up my poop-shoot. I had definitely got beat.

Traveling and pregnancy are imminent high-risk "got beat" situations. An entire litany of bad shit happens to pregnant women, and there's not much you can do to avoid some of the physical discomforts you'll experience. And no doubt it can get in the way of exercising.

Hopefully, you can find a few windows between all the getting beat scenarios during which you can shake that pregnant booty like Beyoncé.

"GOT BEAT" PREGNANCY SIDE EFFECTS

Bloody Gums

Or as my dentist calls it: "Pregnancy Gingivitis." This is very normal and, really, not a big nuisance. And it's (hopefully) temporary. You just get to brush your teeth more often and longer.

Constipation

Yup. This happened to me, and it could be why I got hemorrhoids. Progesterone, the steroid hormone that stimulates the uterus to prepare for pregnancy, is like Xanax for your baby-pushing parts prior to labor. Your uterus muscles need to go on "vacay" so that you don't have contractions ahead of schedule. However, this means your poop-shoot may also hang up its "closed for business" sign. Also, as your baby grows, he can push into your colon and contribute to the "blockage." During a particularly epic bout of constipation, I alternated my "labor" time between the bath, the bed, and the toilet. After five hours, I finally gave birth to the shit. It weighed 4 pounds and measured 5 inches.

Extra Spit

There's no clear explanation as to why this happens, but some people believe it's due to hormones or nausea. I have a co-worker who suffered from this, who had a designated cup on her desk that she spat into like a baseball manager during the World Series. We had to quarantine her in a remote corner of the office.

Hemorrhoids

(Or pesky piles, as the British call them.) These fuckers are puffed-up veins in the anus. Sometimes the blood vessels get so thin and irritated that passing a hard, big stool may be as painful as childbirth. I've torn the crap out of my butthole during some of these "labors." If these swollen veins burst, you may bleed. This can be scary, but these rectal lacerations are usually nothing to fear and quick to heal. Just make sure the blood is coming from the rear.

Itchy Skin

During the third trimester, your belly may be so itchy you'll be tempted to turn it into a scratching pad for Mr. Whiskers. This itchiness, which can spread to your entire body, can be due to dry, stretched skin or to an increased blood supply to the epidermis. However, it's crucial to ask your midwife or OB/GYN to perform a blood screening, because severe itching can also indicate a rare but serious liver disorder called intrahepatic cholestasis of pregnancy (ICP).

Lightning Crotch or Vagina

Sharp bursts of pain to the pelvic area (also known as "fanny daggers") that can even hinder your walking. Typically occurring during the third trimester, causes vary from cervical dilation to Baby changing positions to a magnesium deficiency. One friend said it felt like her baby was gonna fall from between her legs. She had to don a pelvis brace and have a chiropractor "adjust" the area, which involved him sticking his hand you-know-where to crack her pelvic bones. Yikes.

Linea Nigra

No, you're not part zebra or incubating one in your womb. This brown-ish "pregnancy line," up to a half-inch wide, runs from your belly button to the pubic bone. Experts don't know the exact reason for this belly branding but surmise that it's due to hormones—possibly the same hormone that causes your nipples to darken. If it distresses you, cover it up, because there's nothing you can do to make it go away. However, it should disappear on its own after you have your baby.

Pimple Town

Due to all the hormones brewing in your body, you may get acne or bad skin breakouts while pregnant. Fortunately, a few baby-safe products have been created to help you fight these nasty zits, which should never be allowed back after puberty.

Pregnancy Rhinitis

Or as I like to call it: "Snoring Beast." I don't think I snored much, but if a bleeding asshole wasn't enough, my nostrils were bloody pretty much every single day during the nine months I was with child.

Purple Vagina or Chadwick's Sign

This is caused by the change in blood-flow patterns in your nether regions. While ugly, it's not usually a cause for concern. My friend's vajajay reportedly not only changed colors, but her veins protruded Linda-Hamilton-in-*Terminator* style. She probably also had the next "got beat" side effect:

Varicose Vagina or Vulvar Varicose Veins

Due as well to increased blood flow, along with the pelvis being compressed by all the extra weight. Varicose veins can also spread to your thighs and legs. Fun times. But while it may take 3-4 months after you give birth for them to fully disappear, the good news is that, unlike the Terminator, these fuckers won't be back.

Shake That Pregnant Booty

Outside of any "got beat" scenarios, if and when you are able to exercise while pregnant, there are many safe workouts you can do. It's important to select the workout routine that's right for you and to stick with it.

Only you know what type of activity is going to make you happy. And if that's couch-surfing...maybe try leg lifts and bicep curls in front of the tube. Working out is good for you and Baby!

One of the biggest myths I'd like to challenge is that pregnant women shouldn't work out their abs. It's important to strengthen your abdominal wall to help your body carry a growing baby without too much collateral damage. Of course, there are well-known no-no's such as: never do crunches or exercise lying flat on your stomach. But there are many pregnant-appropriate core and abdominal exercises.

For legitimate exercise, I did uphill walks, Pilates, prenatal yoga, and a barre-type class I love called Pop Physique. I also maximized any opportunity in my daily routine to burn calories. I turned tooth-brushing into a sixty-second step-aerobic routine, curled five-pound weights while on the phone at work, and did calf-raises at the gas pump.

I believe good health, genes, and sheer luck helped me sustain my active lifestyle; but conversely, I believe that my active lifestyle helped *me* sustain a healthy pregnancy.

My Favorite Ways to Shake It

Just as the doctor ordered, I kept doing all the exercises I'd enjoyed pre-pregnancy. My go-to workouts included:

WALKING

You put one foot in front of the other, over and over again. It's easier than riding a bicycle, which you *shouldn't* do while pregnant. Walking is relatively kind to your knees and ankles, depending on your weight and the topography you're undertaking. Walking is known to strengthen your heart, help maintain a healthy blood pressure, and improve sleep. Best of all, it's free. All you need is a good pair of kicks.

I've taken urban hikes for as long as I can remember. As a teenager in Guaynabo, Puerto Rico, I trekked along rows of cloned housing in our hilly gated suburban community. During undergrad, I refused to drive to school and instead crossed town lines by stomping down the railroad tracks along the Monongahela River—once, during a pretty heavy storm, only to find out that the university had been snowed out.

So if I could walk through blizzards, why would I let a little fetus stop me?

During my first six months of pregnancy, I continued to drag my ass out of bed before work three to five times a week for a three-mile hike. Mind you, I'm not a morning person, but I'd always been incapable of exercising after a long day at work. (That time was reserved for dining and drinking.) So at first light, I made sure to climb steep hills and stairs, on which I did leg lifts to keep the junk away from my trunk. At the end of my third trimester when my regular routine became unrealistic, I took long strolls around the neighborhood.

YOGA AND PRENATAL YOGA

If you've never been a fan of yoga, pregnancy will most likely not turn you into a yogi. If you are...*Namaste!*

I love yoga and have practiced it on and off for fifteen years. But prenatal yoga was a different story. I felt like a pork chop in a vegan shop around all the beautiful granola mamas-to-be. All the girls in my prenatal classes seemed to *love* being pregnant, trading doula stories and discussing different forms of placenta consumption. Not that there's anything wrong with that—in fact, I almost did both of those things—but the truth is that I am intimidated by earth mamas. Maybe it's because I secretly wish I were more like them.

I never really embraced pregnancy as a beautiful miracle unto itself; I accepted it as a condition that would eventually give me my beautiful miracle. So being around expecting women who were intimately in touch with the ethereal aspect of pregnancy made me feel like I was missing something—some vital aspect of womanhood that I had been born without. For that reason, I favored regular classes, which I frequented on weekends.

Everyone loves to see the knocked-up girl working out, and I admit that being the only pear-bellied chick doing Bakasana (Crow Pose) made me feel like a badass.

There are many benefits to doing yoga while pregnant. Studies show that yoga improves sleep; reduces stress; increases the strength, flexibility, and endurance of muscles needed for childbirth; and decreases lower-back pain and the risk of preterm labor. Prenatal yoga promotes healthy breathing techniques that can help during labor. It also strengthens the pelvic floor.

I did prenatal yoga every weekend up through my forty-first week of pregnancy, when I was as graceful as a circus elephant doing sun salutations. I kept attending because I had heard that in addition to booty blasts, women's waters broke all the time during class. I wanted mine to break because my baby was a little behind schedule. It didn't.

But I did get this out of yoga: During labor, the nurse told me that my hips, inner thighs, and lower back would be sore for days after childbirth. I never felt pain or soreness in any of those areas. I credit both yoga and Pilates for that.

Pelvic Floor: What, Why, and How?

The pelvic floor is like a giant hairball of muscles, ligaments, nerves, and connective tissues attached to the pelvis that aid in the physics of carrying a child, helps with labor, and is primarily responsible for an effective bladder.

It's important to strengthen your pelvic floor before and during pregnancy, because it will get wrecked during vaginal birth. And it's *imperative* to continue working it out afterwards if you want things to go back to normal down there. I mean, those pee-pad panties are great and all, but there's no need to embrace this baby-pushing side effect.

And stop doing the happy dance if you're having a C-section. According to yoga teacher and writer Amy Lynch, "Women who have had Caesareans also need to strengthen their pelvic floor muscles, as it is the gravitational pressure of pregnancy that weakens the muscles, not the physical event of birth" (MindBodyGreen.com, May 2012).

That said, your vagina and labia *will* be spared if you get the C-cut, and I hear that leaking incidents are usually less frequent, indicating that maybe the pelvic floor does gets less "beat" if you have a C-section.

PILATES

Formerly known as "contrology," this exercise designed by German expat Joseph Pilates builds body strength, controlled agility, and flexibility. Since it strengthens your core muscles without straining the joints, it's great for pregnant women. Core muscles encompass your lower back, gluteus, abdominals, and pelvic floor. Since Pilates provides safe ways to target your abs, you can incorporate it if your doctor agrees.

Pilates is key to getting your body up to snuff after delivery. Working out the pelvic floor even helps get your kitty cat back to its pre-childbirth glory—at least, I like to think so (either that, or my husband's lying). Another benefit of Pilates is improved blood circulation. This could reduce leg-swelling and cramping during pregnancy and hopefully prevent a bulbous purple vagina.

I loved my Pilates class, and towards the end when I didn't feel like going out in public (afraid my loose butt cheeks might betray me), I did Pilates at home with Erica Ziel's *Knocked-Up Fitness for the Sassy Modern Mom* DVD. Ziel's got more sweets than sass; she never said anything cheeky when I wobbled, butt-sneezed, or ate through one of her exercises. Plus, I could always turn her off when my husband entered the room. At some point towards the end of pregnancy, I realized that in order to maintain some sort of self-respect, exercise had to be kept private.

DWYCWYC (DO WHAT YOU CAN WHEN YOU CAN)— IT'S NEAT!

I've been practicing this mantra all of my life, but unbeknownst to my social-media-challenged self (I still don't know whether it's pronounced "twit" or "twat" or how the hell hashtags work), two savvy ladies started the hashtag #dwycwyc: "Do What You Can When You Can." So, thank you, ladies, for #branding what I used to refer as "burning calories" and "mini-workouts" back when cell phones were bigger than laptops. And laptops? Well, those weren't even around yet.

The DWYCWYC philosophy goes beyond just cramming a workout into your schedule. It means making exercise a part of everyday life and maximizing every opportunity to burn calories.

I should point out that if you're easily embarrassed, DWYCWYC may not be practical for you. But I don't mind making an arse out of myself in public if it means I get to burn extra calories.

NEAT: NON-EXERCISE ACTIVITY THERMOGENESIS

NEAT is energy we burn while we go about our lives. This includes fidgeting, chewing gum, and annoying, restless "Jimmy legs." All these "moves" can add up to burning 300–2,000 calories a day, depending on your weight, lifestyle, and capacity for gum-chomping.

Examples of DWYCWYC

- While brushing your teeth, do 60 knee lifts. If you have mild to moderate pregnancy gingivitis like I did, do 180.

- After showering, do 30 plié squats while squeezing your palms together for a boob boost.

- Do calf-raises while pumping gas.

- Do butt-clenches when reading or watching TV.

- Do a set of Kegels every time you:

  » See a hot guy.

  » Think sex is on the horizon.

  » Do the dishes.

» Get stuck trying to make a left turn in an intersection. (If you live in L.A., your pussy will be as strong as a Venus flytrap.)

» Pee. Interrupt that stream. It's the best indicator of tightness. The torrential difference between my prepartum and postpartum pee stream was quite depressing.

» Feed your baby. (Yes, in order to get things up to the desired tautness, you need to do Kegels *that* often.)

• Keep weights or resistance bands handy. You can make up an ongoing game with yourself; for example, do a set every time Kerry Washington says "Consider it handled," your boss sends an excruciatingly long passive-aggressive email, or your friend posts her baby yawning on social media.

• Instead of walking to your car, RUN. Okay, this may not be appropriate during the third trimester or with a child in your arms, but it's still one of my favorites. I'm surprised no one has ever come to my rescue, thinking I was being chased. Good ol' Hollywood Boulevard.

• Every time you bend down to pick up something, do a nice squat or plié (or two or three). Make it count, even if it's just one.

• Do lunges across the office on your way to the copier. Who cares what your co-workers think?

• Do counter push-ups (or real ones) in the kitchen while you wait for the microwave.

- Break into a plank every time you have an ice cream craving, and hold it while you sing your favorite song.

- When carrying groceries, do arm curls with the heavy bags—I learned that one from my dad.

- When you're clear to work out after childbirth, break every hour or so and do burpees. (Google it: XHIT Daily's "How to Do a Burpee" tutorial video has over five million hits on YouTube.)

Other Workouts and Safety Tips

Besides the workouts and activities already discussed, other safe workouts include swimming, kayaking, jogging, and spinning. Swimming is great because there's no impact to the joints and the water helps carry your weight while you do laps. And yeah, stationary biking is safe, but its only advisable if you're already a "spinner"; taking up spinning or running while pregnant is not recommended.

If CrossFit is your jam, safe and specific workouts for pregnant women have been developed. Though why anyone besides Conan the Barbarian would want to pull a tire across a parking lot is beyond my comprehension-bandwidth. (*Oops.* Just found out my editor digs this kind of stuff. Sorry, Jennifer!)

If you're a hard-core runner or a boot-camp biatch, you can probably still engage in some activity as long as you keep it fairly low impact and avoid lying on your stomach.

Doctors also recommend you avoid lying on your back because of the pressure the baby puts on your intestines and your major blood vessels, the aorta and vena cava. (And I thought cava was Spain's champagne!) But your doctor may allow you to do so for short periods if it's comfortable.

Safety DOs And DON'Ts
for Exercising While Pregnant

DO be aware of your "swollen" sense of gravity; a pregnant belly can mess up your balance, so mind the bump. (I was going for a pun on the U.K.'s metro system, but it didn't quite work.)

DON'T walk in extremely hot weather. It's very easy to overheat when you're pregnant, so bring plenty of water to hydrate and plan a route with shaded areas or coffee shops so you can sit down and take a break. This is a good time to exercise vocal chords and catch up with the fam.

DO take it easy and work out at a comfortable pace. Getting thirsty, very tired, or lightheaded isn't good for Mom or Baby.

DON'T overdo it. Pregnancy is not the time to "push" that extra set. Save it for the delivery room. When I felt the reps were too many or didn't feel comfortable with a technique, I modified or rested. Sometimes I did Kegels instead (which, by the way, may be a wives' tale I took a chance on; there's no real evidence that doing them before labor lessens the impact childbirth has on the pelvic muscles).

BIG
NO-NO!

Danger Signs

If you experience any of the following symptoms, stop whatever you're doing and call your doctor at once:

- **Chest pain**
- **Vaginal bleeding**
- **Calf-swelling or pain**
- **Amniotic fluid leakage**
- **Contractions**

BIG
NØ-NØ!

Do Not Attempt While Pregnant

While pregnant, avoid the following types of activities:

- Sports that involve a fast-moving object*

- High-contact sports**

- Sports that challenge gravity***

- Changing cat litter (cat shit can transmit a hazardous parasite)

Examples:

* Tennis (unless you're Serena Williams), Dodge Ball, Baseball, Softball, Volleyball, Racquetball, Basketball, Soccer, Paintball, Hockey

** Martial Arts, Wrestling, Kickboxing, Boxing, Football, Rugby, Roller Derby

*** Surfing, Snowboarding, Mountain Biking, Gymnastics, any kind of Skiing or Skating, Rock Climbing

If you wish to remain active through your pregnancy, consult an expert to help you choose a fitness routine that suits your lifestyle.

While exercising, the most important thing is to listen to your body. Learn through my embarrassing example.

Who Let the Farts Out?

When you can no longer hold your own gas, it's time to quit group classes. The wind was too sleek and my butt cheeks too slow. I didn't know what was happening until it was right at the threshold. It was loud and distinct, but people pretended not to hear it. Oh, but you know they did! The unspoken etiquette on cutting the cheese is simple: culprits and victims completely ignore the noise and/ or smell. Thankfully, my ass acoustics didn't come with an aroma. Quick aside: Why is it that the stench of your own "cheesy puffs" doesn't really make you double over in disgust? You know it stinks, but you keep whiffing, trying to dissect the new scent line coming out of your anus. *Was that the beer, the bean burrito, or the brussels sprouts? Regardless, I hope nobody walks in on me right now.*

Situation "stinker alert" aside, it became challenging to do anything with a nine-month-pregnant belly, a.k.a. bodily function piñata. Pee, fart, and shart...one misstep and out came one, two, or all of the above. And if you're blushing at this, get used to it. Because gross stuff like this will happen to you very often from now on. But if you look good, people may be more disposed to forgive the yuck-factor. (I know it's unfair, but I didn't make the rules.)

Working Out After Baby

As a new mom, making time to get out of the house and away from my baby was difficult, but it was key to retaining my mental health. Getting back to my pre-pregnancy figure gave me strength and confidence—two things every good mom needs.

After assessing your body's well-being and with your doctor's go-ahead, you can safely resume working out as early as two weeks after a vaginal birth. Most doctors recommend you wait six weeks after a C-section. I eased into Pilates on week three and slowly built back up. By week six, I was back at Pop Physique. Of course, I almost yelled: "Can I get an epidural over here?" during some of the exercises. Sadly, that wasn't an option.

In all seriousness, getting fit is empowering. This is true for any passion worth pursuing. No question it's hard to find time, but it's also easy to use the lack of time, sleep, and help as excuses. You don't even have to call in the sitter or negotiate with your partner to watch the baby; you can find short, free workouts online that you can cram in when your baby isn't crawling yet. Once baby is on the move, put her in an exersaucer while *you* exercise. You can even make it "entertainment" time: she'll love to watch you move. Another good Mommy and Me exercise is taking your baby for a walk or jog. You can get a great workout just from pushing that jogger or stroller uphill (just make sure your baby is IN it. Otherwise, that would be weird).

When I got back to work, cramming in a session became more difficult. Coffee sprints and mini-workout breaks sprinkled through the day were all I could do until the weekends, when I carved time to "move," even if it was power walking at the mall with my baby in the Bjorn.

The commitment to exercise does wane, the busier (and more exhausted) you become and the more children you have. It's hard enough as it is!

And as previously discussed, it may take time to get back to your pre-pregnancy weight—if ever. However, if you feel you're doing everything you can but don't see results, consult a fitness expert and/or a nutritionist.

Finally, commiserating woman-to-woman: Even after all these workouts, I *still* pee myself a little when I cough, sneeze, or laugh real hard. Got beat is right.

SEX, LIES, AND MASTURBATE

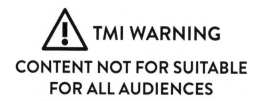

Your Lady Parts Deserve R&R

⚠ **TMI WARNING**

**CONTENT NOT FOR SUITABLE
FOR ALL AUDIENCES**

If you're the father of my child, my parents, or most importantly, my in-laws: PLEASE DO EVERYBODY A FAVOR AND SKIP TO THE NEXT CHAPTER. Seriously, Cathy, this means YOU.

I'M HAPPY TO REPORT that many women feel quite passionate throughout their pregnancies and enjoy bumping uglies with an actual bump. But for me, sex while seven-plus months pregnant sucks dick—and you may have to do a lot of that just to avoid vaginal penetration. Or do a whole lot of nothing if your gag reflexes worsen with your baby pushing against your esophagus.

But don't worry: dry-heaving, morning sickness, and hemorrhoids permitting, you can enjoy a healthy sex life through your first trimester and a good chunk of your second. It's only the last two months that suck. Love those puns.

During the early months, you'll still be able to explore every position in the *Kama Sutra* and enjoy all stages of foreplay if you're feeling up to it. And that's a big *IF* because sometimes nausea or the big ol' brain will get in the way of sexy times. Physically, your growing bump will inevitably get in the way of missionary work. Safe and simple positions are spooning, crab, forward-facing cowgirl, reverse cowgirl, scissors, edge of the bed, doggie-style, and the policeman (pretend you're being frisked against the wall). You can also use pillows, props, and a vivid imagination to play out whatever fantasy works for you and your partner.

> "I had forgotten about the pregnancy sex dreams. Whoa, mama."
>
> —S.M.T., Executive, Los Angeles, CA,
> *Pregnant with #2*

If you can ride your man, full-belly on top and love it, I want to commemorate you on my tombstone. Seriously. I'm too self-conscious for that rodeo. The only way for me to enjoy sex was to ignore the pregnant belly in the room. I had to face it away from my partner and then close my eyes so I wouldn't have to look at it either.

As my bump grew, my options shrank: reverse cowgirl required too much work on my part and policeman was not comfortable—the pressure of my belly on my pelvis wouldn't tolerate it. So that narrowed it down to doggie-style and spoon-style. Then, it got worse. Towards the last month, when the colony of hemorrhoids pollinated my anus, there was no way I was giving my husband front-row seats to the new kids on the block. Doggie-style was sent to the doghouse.

So faithful spoon-style took us through the last two weeks. Yup. We made it. I wanted to make it. It brought me relief and pride to complete the operational mission of providing my husband with a "place to put it." Sex is intimacy. And that's my favorite part about it.

Sex made me feel like I was desired and gave me a way to connect with my beloved husband, who is right now probably trying to figure out if over-sharing stands up in court as valid grounds for divorce.

Pregnant Sex: Safety Guidelines

It's safe to have sex and masturbate while pregnant, unless your doctor advises you against it for medical reasons. Most standard sexual practices will not cause a miscarriage or hurt your baby. Your fetus is protected by the amniotic fluid in your uterine muscles. (If you're into dirty talk, try to whisper "uterus" and "amniotic fluid" in your partner's ear to move things along.)

There are just a few warnings to heed while engaging in pregnant bed sports:

○ Even though you don't have to worry about pregnancy, if you're heterosexual and not in a monogamous or STD-free relationship, you'll need a slipper for that Cinderella. In addition to your own personal discomfort, having a herpes outbreak during vaginal delivery can be detrimental to your baby's health.

○ Anal sex followed by vaginal intercourse is never advisable. Your A-hole could house bacteria that you don't want in your V-hole. This could lead to a urinary tract infection, ranging from cystitis to pyelonephritis, a serious kidney infection. If you're into this combo, wear a different condom for each orifice and/or clean up between penetrations.

○ Some precautionary advice also exists against receiving oral sex. (I know...why couldn't it be against giving it?!) There's a chance your partner could unintentionally blow an air bubble up your vagina while going down on you. It rarely happens, but this burst of air could block a blood vessel and cause an air embolism, which could be life-threatening to your child. Try explaining that to your in-laws.

BIG
NØ-NØ!

Avoid Sex If...

- You have unexplained vaginal bleeding.

- You are leaking amniotic fluid (rush to see your doctor if you suspect this).

- Your cervix is opening prematurely (your doctor should be keeping tabs on it during checkups).

- You suffer from placenta previa (your placenta partly or completely covers your cervical opening).

- You have a history of preterm labor (although research in this area has been deemed limited and biased, so heed at your own discretion).

If none of the big no-nos applies to you and you're in the mood, sex it up—because after baby you'll have to be abstinent for six weeks.

My Cosmo-Worthy Sex Tips

In the words of Alec Baldwin in *Outside Providence:* "Making sex is like a Chinese dinner: It ain't over 'til you both get your cookies." So. How do you get your cookie?

#1 *Think of your pussy*

And you have to call it that in order to get into the right headspace. You can't think about what to make for dinner, or that your bunched-up thigh against the bed looks like Slimer from *Ghostbusters,* or how Carrie will survive her current predicament in *Homeland.* To bring your O into *your* homeland, you must concentrate on the good feeling happening in your lady parts.

#2 *Choose your own fantasy*

Peruse your spank-bank. Remember when sex used to be longer and hotter? You can teleport you and your partner into the bleachers of your old school. Or imagine you're the hot sitter and the wife's coming home. Or fantasize you're bound. Those are mine. Feel free to steal 'em.

#3 *Live out that fantasy*

Getting tied up in bed isn't that difficult. Have fun with your surroundings. Wear a blindfold or a sexy nurse costume. Go sit on your partner's desk while he's at the computer and refuse to leave until he does as he's told. Whatever rocks your boat. "Do it" and have fun with it.

#4 *Masturbate*

It doesn't have to be elaborate. You don't need a warm bath, candles, and soft music. Like an adolescent, rubbing up against a rolled-up sock will do. Porn works well, too. Or you can dust off old Mr. Rabbit and put him to good use. All you need is an efficient, connect-the-dots affair that bears no casualties or witnesses.

Dude, I really hope my MIL is not reading this!

#5 *Think outside traditional sex lines*

Sex isn't limited to vaginal penetration. This is particularly important after giving birth, when your vagina isn't up to snuff or your C-section scar is still healing. You can do oral, dry hump, enter through the rear, engage in manual labor...even rubbing up against thighs, knees, and buttocks can achieve the same goal: climaxing.

#6 *Don't underestimate first base*

Many men and women need genital separation during pregnancy and/or after birth. This is perfectly normal. In time, you will get back on the proverbial horse. There's no need to rush to the finish line.

However, finding ways to connect physically during particularly dry spells, be it through gentle touches, cuddling, spooning, kissing, foot massages, hand-holding, or even a spontaneous hug, can really make a positive difference in a relationship. Skin-on-skin contact is not just for baby.

Sex After Baby

Vaginal labor is like playing the lottery with your Lady V: You can win the unsullied prize, or it can take years to feel normal down there—way longer than the recommended six-week abstinence period.

Unless you had a fairly severe vaginal or labia tear, recovery from vaginal labor is similar to that of a C-section. We all suffer from postpartum bleeding and must wait for our uteruses to shrink and our cervixes to close up. Not to mention all the psychological mumbo jumbo that follows having a kid. We all bear scars, both literally and metaphorically.

However, I do think that women who pushed out a baby have it worse when it comes to resuming lovemaking. For some of us, the prescribed post-delivery abstinence may be a relief. *Will my lady parts ever recover from this extraction?* I remember wondering.

And the first time? The first time hurts like a motherfucker. Having sex after vaginal birth is almost as frightening as taking that first shit. You have to psych yourself up for it, relax, and then take it one stride at a time. Literally. Things (or body parts, rather) will slide right into place with a bit of help from your KY friend.

Lubricant is often necessary for either type of birth mama because low levels of estrogen may turn your vajayjay into a dry well—in addition to the "well" still possibly undergoing repair.

For me, it took two months for it to feel good and eight months for it to be better than ever. I had a particular spot (my doctor said it was scar tissue) that really hurt upon penetration. It's possible to get scar tissue from a tear or an episiotomy, and this may cause pain or discomfort during sex. In my experience with this, it only ached "at the gate." After that initial "ouch," everything felt great.

It takes a while to get back on the healthy sex-life track, as many factors are involved beyond the healing of the traumatized region. For reasons raging from body image to hormones, it may be harder to get in the mood or feel as sexual as you did before baby—especially when the process has done to your body what a shredder does to paper. Heck, during the first year, your exhaustion alone may be reason enough to have a sex therapist on speed dial.

Most couples tend to go through dry and wet spells regardless of whether or not they just had a baby. After a baby, the loss of libido is even more common, for both men and women. And if you're breastfeeding, the hormone prolactin may inhibit your sex drive. Not to mention you may fear spraying breast milk all over the place. As a precaution, I had sex in my crispy nursing bra for a year after I had my daughter. Super sexy times.

In contrast to the abundance of women's stories after giving birth, there is a dearth of relevant information on a man's libido after witnessing childbirth. But I hunted some down.

"I truly believe couples would have more chance of normal intimacy after a birth if men saw less of the delivery," writes father and husband Martin Daubney (*Daily Mail U.K.,* October 2012). "Witnessing childbirth—the most intimate experience in life—leaves a lasting impression on a man [that] can drive a wedge between himself and his wife."

Martin blamed his loss of libido on witnessing the pain his wife suffered during a very long complicated labor that ended in a C-section. He felt guilty. But there are more shallow reasons, too. Like watching a woman pump or breastfeed. My husband did not like to see that, and I can't judge him for it. He can't help how his body or mind reacts to things like his wife's nipples oozing milk.

Unfortunately, there's no secret sauce that will spruce up libido or magic words that can boost confidence. It takes communication, acceptance, and effort from both parties to resume a healthy sex life after Baby. It's important to address the elephant in the bedroom. The road to sexual normalcy has a bumpy start, but with a bit of effort, you can get back in the saddle.

After my scar tissue went away, sex became beyond amazing. It could be that I forgot how good it used to be before pregnancy, or that all those Kegels finally paid off. But I've never enjoyed it this much. I truly credit this fucking miracle to the fucking miracle that is my child (see what I did there?). When she allows us the time and the energy to fuck, I know I'd better get my cookie before that baby starts crying again. She has unwittingly shortened the race to the finish line and made her mom a short-distance, sprint-running champion.

MY GREEN ALTER-MAMA

Baby Steps Towards
a Healthier Home and Womb

THE GRASS IS ALWAYS GREENER on the other side of the fence—which is where my raw-vegan neighbor grows organic vegetables outside her solar-powered home in composted biodegradable diaper liners. She makes cashew butter from scratch, wears organic-cotton free-trade panties, and cleans her baby's nursery with lemon, vinegar, and baking soda. In case you've forgotten, I live in Hippie-fornia.

My side of the railing is a concrete wasteland. I use vinegar to soothe my hands when I burn them baking frozen zucchini fries for my daughter...which is every other day. I'm obsessed with Pampers Swaddlers (they have a line that indicates whether or not your baby needs a change!), was cursed with a black thumb (my cacti have barely survived it), and our gas provider shamed me for how much of it we consume. I take long, hot showers almost every day and, up until recently, bought bottled water in bulk. Moving towards filtered tap water was a baby step towards the green road.

But it felt like a giant stride.

It Ain't Easy Being Green

Being green is a big commitment, and at times I've been a terrible partner. Take, for example, my diaper offense. My daughter took more than ten shits a day—no joke. Washing cloth diapers was not "sustainable"—for me or the environment. I took comfort in knowing that washing diapers accounts for approximately 5 percent of a water bill and that had I signed up for a diaper pickup/wash service, I would've increased my carbon footprint. But although this helped me sleep at night, deep down I knew the truth: We will be buried in trash someday unless we figure out a way to safely dump it on another planet.

After three months of sour soft-serve poop and disposables, I still could've gone green. But by then I was a Swaddlers junkie. And my baby never had a diaper rash during this stage, no matter what cloth diaper activists tell you. But that's just me being defensive: cloth or hybrids are best for Earth *and* Baby.

In order to make up for all the years it will take for my daughter's diapers to decompose, I try to be green in other ways. Because in spite of my transgressions, I love our planet. And I want my life and my daughter's to be healthier, too.

When I was pregnant, I set out to create a healthy environment for my baby inside my body *and* my home. I knew that building a better ecosystem in my womb involved exercising, eating well, and avoiding toxins, so I embarked on figuring out what the heck lived in the dust I breathed and the food I ate, and what—if anything— crossed the placenta and reached my unborn child. Turns out, lots of stuff.

What Toxins Are in My Home and Womb?

Toxicologists are still researching the long-term impact that various compounds have on our babies and us. And most studies are based on laboratory animals or on adults who have experienced an indeterminate amount of prolonged exposure. Still, pretty solid evidence exists that toxins do cross the placenta and affect a fetus.

Studies have discovered chemicals such as perchlorate, bisphenol (BPA), lead, mercury, cadmium, and DDT (a banned pesticide) in amniotic fluid, umbilical cord blood, and infants' first stools. In fact, 232 toxic chemicals were found in umbilical cord blood from U.S. newborns according to a chart published by the Environmental Defense Fund. Some of these substances can be rather destructive to a developing fetus. A toxin that could barely harm an adult could irreparably affect a baby's DNA.

To be clear: Heating up one TV dinner encased in BPA-based plastic and eating it while pregnant is probably not going to harm your fetus. But the studies are stacking up that say long-term exposure to toxins really *can* make a dent in our bodies and our babies, so to speak. So why not, when possible, try to avoid them? It's not only good for you and Baby, but the environment benefits as well. Everyone wins.

My green alter-mama compiled a general cheat sheet of "suspicious" toxins. Depending on the length and frequency of exposure to each, Baby and/or Mom could be impacted by side effects.

THE TOXIC TABLE

toxin	the skinny	where found	potential side effects (to Baby and/or Mom)
BPA (bisphenol A)	A synthetic compound used to harden plastics. Also often used in food cans and packaging to lengthen product shelf life.	• Canned food • Plastic-packaged food and beverages (plastic labeled 3, 6, or 7) • Sippy cups • Baby bottles • Plastic toys • Medical equipment • Receipt paper • CDs and DVDs • Water pipeline	• Increased susceptibility to cancer in utero • Impaired fetal brain development • Impeded genital development and prostate cancer in male babies • Harmful long-term hormone response, and breast development in female babies • Reduced egg quality for moms undergoing in vitro • Obesity

toxin	the skinny	where found	potential side effects (to Baby and/or Mom)
flame retardants	Chemicals added to foam and fabric to make them fire-resistant. These can accumulate in your body and pervade your breast milk, and Baby's cord blood while in utero.	• Furniture • Car upholstery • Baby clothes (particularly pajamas) • Strollers • Car seats • Nursing pillows • Cell phones • TV remotes	• Thyroid disruption • Mental and physical developmental delays • Cognitive problems • Early onset of puberty • Reduced brain development
formaldehyde	Famously known for its use as an embalming fluid, this gas made by oxidizing methanol falls under the Volatile Organic Compound class.	• Glue • Wood by-products (i.e., plywood) • Soaps and detergents • Air fumes	• Inflammation of respiratory airways • Nose cancer • Myeloid leukemia
PCBs (*polychlorinated biphenyls*)	A group of over 200 man-made chemicals, used mainly as flame retardants, many of which have been banned since 1977 but still contaminate our environment.	• High-fat beef and fish	• Non-Hodgkin lymphoma (NHL) • Low birthweight • Developmental delays • Reduced conception rates • Delays in visual recognition • Short-term memory delays

THE TOXIC TABLE (CONT.)

toxin	the skinny	where found	potential side effects (to Baby and/or Mom)
pesticides	Toxins created to kill living organisms. Who the hell wants that shit around their baby?	• Produce • Lawn, garden, and home products	• Leukemia • Lymphoma • Genital abnormalities • Spina bifida • Hydrocephaly
PFCs (perfluorinated compounds)	Fluorine-loaded chemicals that make stuff stain- and stick-resistant.	• Nonstick cookware • Cosmetics • Clothing • Food containers • Carpets • Couches • Dental floss • Nail polish • Moisturizers	• Kidney cancer • High cholesterol • Obesity • Low sperm count • Low birthweight • Abnormal thyroid function
phthalate	A chemical that makes plastic bendable and is often used in fragrances.	• Scented hygiene products (including baby products) • Nail polish • Packaged food • Vinyl tile • Wood varnishes • Cleaning products • Hard plastics • Flexible plastics (i.e., inflatable toys)	• Boys' reproductive development in utero • Impaired fertility in boys • Early puberty in girls • Breast and testicular cancer

Mr. Green Will See You Now

The table above invited you to dip your toes in the eco-pool. If you feel like taking a paddle, here's some more extensive information on the chemicals outlined in the toxic table.

But I can't stress this enough: You can't afford to lose much-needed sleep over this. No one can fully avoid every little thing that could be harmful, so there's no sense losing our minds trying to eliminate exposure to all toxins. However, we can improve our home health by tackling some of the things that are easy for us to modify.

BPA OR BISPHENOL A

Bisphenol A is an endocrine disruptor that "disrupts" normal hormone functioning by mimicking estrogen and decreasing testosterone. BPAs are used to make hard plastic and the lining in food cans. Thankfully, our bodies expunge this chemical fairly quickly, so a little bit of BPA isn't going to kill you. Studies have concluded that the risk is proportionate to the degree of exposure.

Why is this shit bad for me and my baby?

Deemed a "reproductive toxicant," BPA is something we want to keep off our uterus before conceiving and while pregnant. BPAs can cause harm to the baby's own reproductive system and lead to certain types of cancer down the line.

How to avoid?

- 🌍 Avoid canned food except those marked with BPA-free lining. With pain in my heart, I've stopped buying Campbell's Tomato Soup. My grilled cheese will forever miss its BFF. (Though Amy's Cream of Tomato Soup does hold a candle to it and their cans' linings do not contain BPAs.)

- 🌍 Buy fresh ingredients, fresh-frozen foods, and food packaged in glass or TetraPak (box-type containers).

- 🌍 Replace plastic bottles, sippy cups, and food storage containers with glass, silicone, porcelain, or non-insulated stainless steel (make sure the product is 100 percent lead-free). Some newer studies indicate that other harmful chemicals have been used to replace the BPA in BPA-free fare, so if you want to be extra safe, avoid these, too.

- 🌀 Don't microwave anything in plastic or under plastic wrap, as the heat allows the chemicals to leach into the food. Furthermore, don't transfer hot liquids into plastic containers, as the chemicals are still prone to seep into the liquid this way.

FLAME RETARDANTS
(PBDES A.K.A. POLYBROMINATED DIPHENYL ETHERS)

Flame retardants are chemicals added to foam and fabric that have been formulated to prevent fire from spreading. Depending on the size of a piece of furniture, its foam filling may contain several pounds of flame retardants.

I'm sure those who invented this substance had good intentions, but recent studies show that flame retardants may release hydrogen cyanide during a fire, along with other toxic gases, which is the number one cause of death in fires (as fumes usually kill a person before the fire does).

Why is this shit bad for me and my baby?

Flame retardants have been linked to cancer and could impair the liver, kidneys, brain, and testes. Over time, these chemicals build up in the fat in our bodies, and they have been found in breast milk, body fat, infant cord blood, and children's blood.

Particularly interesting is that one study found that the concentration of this chemical was nearly five times higher in children than in their mothers. This is likely because flame retardants aren't chemically bonded to foam or fabric, so the molecules travel freely through the environment our babies crawl around in; these chemicals live in dust and can get into our bodies fairly easy. Just thinking about how much time my daughter spends climbing on the couch gives me the creeps. A new flame-retardant-free couch is on my wish list.

How to avoid?

- 🌐 Seek an all-natural or organic crib mattress. (More on mattress selection in *Chapter 7: Seriously.: How Much Crap Does a Teeny-Weeny Little Baby Need?*)

- 🌐 When furnishing your nursery, find furniture and items that are free of flame retardants.

- 🌐 Purchase baby clothes and blankets made out of organic fibers.

- 🌐 Get rid of your old couch, as they release the most PBDEs. Thanks to revised regulations on flame-retardant chemicals, a lot of companies now manufacture upholstery furniture without flame retardants.

- 🌐 Frequently vacuum your couch.

- 🌐 Wash hands often to avoid ingesting these chemicals or rubbing in your eyes.

FORMALDEHYDE

Formaldehyde is a widely known toxin—perhaps one we've been hearing about since we were little kids (unlike the "millennial" BPAs). According to its definition, formaldehyde is a colorless pungent gas made by oxidizing methanol, whose name derives from formic acid and aldehyde. Formaldehyde falls under the Volatile Organic Compound (VOC) class.

But before we continue our discussion, it's important to note that our bodies produce small, harmless amounts of formaldehyde; therefore, it's not possible—or vital—to completely eliminate it.

Why is this shit bad for me and my baby?

VOCs may be the worst offenders in contributing to poor indoor air quality. Breathing regular doses of formaldehyde may trigger inflammation of the respiratory airways, throat, and eyes. People who suffer from asthma should be particularly careful, as it can set off attacks. High formaldehyde exposure has also been linked to cancer of the nose and myeloid leukemia.

After Hurricane Katrina hit in 2005, many people housed in FEMA-issued trailers suffered from respiratory difficulties, nosebleeds, and headaches. This was allegedly caused by high doses of off-gas emanating from the furniture. Think a hotbox of formaldehyde.

How to avoid?

- If you work at a manufacturing company and are exposed to high levels of this substance, talk to your employer about ways to minimize your exposure, or explore opportunities in safer work environments.

- Purchase wood by-products labeled "CARB phase 2 compliance" or stick to solid wood.

- Air out wood by-products before taking them inside the house.

- Air out your home often if you have a lot of particle-wood furniture or laminate floor.

PCBS

Polychlorinated biphenyls are very hearty man-made chlorinated chemicals once used in many products, such as coolants, insulating fluids, plasticizers in paints and cements, and PVC coatings.

PCBs are now banned due to health concerns, but these chemicals are like cockroaches: They're hard to eliminate from the environment. They live in our soil, water, and air. The fish, meat, dairy, and produce we consume hail from those three elements. Therefore, we may take in PCBs through inhalation, skin absorption, and ingestion.

Since PCBs are not easily broken down, they accumulate in our bodies. PCBs amass in animal fat and are most commonly found in fish. Reference the Push Tip on the opposite page for further details on picking the healthiest fish to eat.

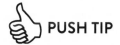 **PUSH TIP**

Selecting the Least-Toxic Fish

- For bigger fish fare, wild-caught tuna and salmon are usually less polluted. I prefer Alaskan or Scottish salmon.

- Other fish low in PCBs are herring, sardines, crappie, yellow perch, and bluegills.

- Bottom-feeders such as catfish, buffalo fish, and carp are usually high in PCBs.

- Very large fish such as walleye and bass tend to eat the aforementioned bottom-feeders, thereby ingesting PCBs.

- Avoid fish from highly polluted rivers such as the Hudson.

- Avoid or be very discerning when selecting farm-raised fish and shrimp. Very often, farm-raised salmon is fattened with corn (ever heard of a fish wanting to eat corn?) and seafood pellets that contain colorants to give the fish that "rosy" glow.

Why is this shit bad for me and my baby?

Like most widely available pollutants, occasional exposure to PCBs is not correlated with major health issues. However, PCBs are probable human carcinogens and endocrine disruptors. PCBs affect the reproductive, endocrine, nervous, and immune systems. And because they mess with our hormones, it's particularly important to avoid while pregnant. PCBs have been linked as a risk factor to non-Hodgkin's lymphoma. They can also affect thyroid hormone levels.

How to avoid?

- ⊕ Wash hands and faces often—especially after playing with dirt.

- ⊕ Buy wild, pole-caught fish, be discerning when choosing farm-raised fare and avoid bottom-feeders. *(Reference Push Tip: Selecting the Least-Toxic Fish.)*

- ⊕ Use and endorse organic, grass-fed and finished, low-fat poultry, meat, and dairy. PCBs tend to accumulate in fatty tissue.

PESTICIDES

Many farmers resort to pesticides to keep animals off their crops (including cotton fields). Their crops absorb this poison and we consume it (or wear it). Pesticides also travel with wind and rain, settling in urban homes. Experts approximate that the median household hosts about three to ten gallons of toxic materials. So, it is virtually impossible to live free and clear of pesticides. But we can minimize our exposure to it.

Why is this shit bad for me and my baby?

Weed killers and pesticides may cause cancer, particularly leukemia and lymphoma as outlined above. Expectant moms should avoid working in pesticide-friendly facilities at all costs, for risk of affecting their fetus's neurological system, especially when exposed to high doses.

Some studies further indicate a relationship between pesticides and ADHD, and even autism. "Last year, researchers at the MIND (Medical Investigation of Neurodevelopmental Disorders) Institute reported that pregnant women who lived near fields where chemical pesticides were used had a roughly two-thirds higher risk of having a child with autism spectrum disorder, and even higher risk of having one with other developmental delays" (Ginny Graves, *Parents Magazine,* p. 134, December 2015).

This high-pesticide environment has also been associated with genital abnormalities in boys, and chronic exposure to certain pesticides has been connected with birth defects like spina bifida, hydrocephaly (excess cranial fluid resulting in an enlarged skull), shortened limbs, and lower IQ scores in children, and with poor semen quality and endometriosis in adults.

How to avoid?

- Buy organic produce. According to the American Cancer Society, nonorganic food doesn't increase the risk of cancer; however, organic food is, for the most part, pesticide-free.

- Scrub produce with water or a plant-based cleaner to wash off chemicals.

- Choose organic cotton and other natural fabrics.

- Reduce or rid your home and garden of pesticides and herbicides.

- Remove your shoes at the door to prevent tracking chemicals into your home.

- Use and endorse all-natural products to eradicate household pests. For example:

  - Boric acid helps get rid of fleas, ants, silverfish, and cockroaches. It also has antifungal properties.

  - Eucalyptus leaves and diffused essential oils such as citronella may keep insects at bay.

  - Peppermint oil is said to keep mice away.

  - Squirting cayenne pepper diluted in oil could help keep squirrels away from your trees.

  - Adopt a cat.

PFCS

Also known as Perfluorinated Compounds, PFCs are like PCBs: vermin that are ridiculously hard to kill. Because they accumulate in the environment, you can also find PFCs in water sources, fish, and livestock—especially near PFC manufacturing plants. PFCs leak from factories and are in consumer products such as nonstick cookware. They also collect in dust. We all probably have traces of PFCs in our blood. Scientists still don't know if it can be absorbed through the skin.

The most common forms of PFCs are PFOA (perfluorooctanoic acid) used to make Teflon products and PFOS (perfluorooctane sulfonate) formerly used in Scotchguard products. I'm in the process of replacing all my nonstick cookware with cast iron or ceramic. It's a costly endeavor, but we're slowly chipping away at this goal.

Why is this shit bad for me and my baby?

Since our bodies don't easily eliminate these toxins, frequent exposure to PFCs over time allows them to accumulate in our brain, liver, lungs, bones, muscles, and kidneys, which can be detrimental to our health. PFCs have been known to cross the placenta barrier and have been found in breast milk.

How to avoid?

- Replace nonstick cookware with ceramic or cast iron. If this is not feasible, at least try to not heat the pan to over 450°F.
- Discard nonstick pots with a deteriorated coating or scratch marks.
- If you live in an area where your water supply could be compromised, drink purified water and install filters in your water taps and shower.
- Abstain from microwaving popcorn bags and frozen pizza (that silver "microwaveable" lining is *no bueno*).
- Avoid stain-resistant finishes on furniture and upholstery.

PHTHALATES

Saying phthalates may trip your tongue, but these chemicals are what make plastic bendable. They are also used in some fragrances. And like PCBs, phthalates can be inhaled, ingested, or absorbed through the skin.

Certain workplace environments, such as the automotive industry, rubber-hose manufacturing facilities, and nail salons, are "richer" in this toxin.

Why is this shit bad for me and my baby?

Like BPAs and PCBs, phthalates are endocrine-disruptive and should be avoided while pregnant. The endocrine system produces the hormones that regulate metabolism, growth and development, tissue function, sexual function, reproduction, sleep, and mood. These are all crucial to our bodies, which is why endocrine disruptors can be so dangerous to a developing fetus. Studies have connected reduced testosterone levels, lowered sperm counts, genital defects, and impaired fertility with exposure to phthalates and other endocrine disruptors while in utero.

How to avoid?

- Since BPA and phthalates can be found in plastic containers, abstaining from microwaving in plastic is an easy yet big step towards improving your body's well-being.

- Write off Plastic #3. It's particularly loaded with phthalates.

- Look for cleaning products and toys that are plant-based, BPA-free, and phthalate-free. Specifically toys that your baby will want to put in his mouth. Also, be mindful of toys coated with lead paint.

- Go fragrance-free. There are just too many chemicals in synthetic fragrances. Natural fragrances are usually safe. (Usually, because "all-natural" is not always a reliable endorsement. Not all chemicals are bad and not all natural things are good. Isn't the oleander plant poisonous?)

- Avoid or limit chemical cleaning supplies. Distilled white vinegar diluted in water (with, if you like, a little bit of lemon essential oil) is a great way to kill most household germs and keep your counters clean. However, when it comes time to clean the diaper bin, I go straight for the disinfectant; but I spray the bin outdoors and let it air out before putting it back in our daughter's room.

- 🌍 Avoid purchasing products that contain phthalates. DBP, DEP, DEHP, BIs, BzBP, DMP are all phthalates to be avoided.
- 🌍 Choose plastics with the recycling code 1, 2, 4, or 5.
- 🌍 Avoid products with recycling codes 3, 6, and 7, as they probably contain phthalates (or BPA).

50 Shades of Peroxide

Traditional hair dyes may contain chemicals such as phthalates and formaldehyde. However, the APA deems hair dye safe for pregnant women because the amount of chemicals absorbed through the system is too minimal to pose a threat for Baby.

General recommendations include postponing processing until after the first trimester, using semi-permanent dyes, avoiding bleaching or stripping prior to dyeing, and seeking henna, organic, and/or vegetable-based dyes.

This was one instance when I took a calculated risk because I couldn't allow myself to walk around with gray strays for *too* long. Thankfully, my situation wasn't dire; so during my entire pregnancy, I was able to make do with only one root touch-up after my first trimester using semi-permanent color.

There are other dyes that I *did* choose to avoid.

The Tint—and Taint—of Food Dyes

Dyes are widely used in processed foods, drinks, and condiments to—you guessed it—*dye* the food to make it look more appealing. Think glow-in-the-dark mac 'n' cheese.

The U.S. doesn't regulate the use of synthetic food dyes, most of which are derived from petroleum. Conversely, countries like the U.K. require food companies to display warning labels on their packaging if their product contains artificial colors. In order to avoid posting a warning label, the same company makes a dye-free version of their product available only in the U.K.; the U.S. version still contains dye. Effed up, right?

The research on food dyes isn't bulletproof, but artificial food dyes may contain carcinogens and have been linked to behavioral problems in children. Because of these findings, parents have begun to avoid artificial dyes and have reported positive changes in their children's behaviors.

Thankfully, food manufacturers are listening, and they're finding wholesome alternatives to food dyes. Don't be afraid to be that person in the aisle reading labels. At the top of the most wanted list are Red #40, Yellow #5, and Yellow #6.

Below is a chart outlining the bright suspects that have been connected to specific side effects. Some of their names sound like superheroes. Don't be fooled.

TO-DYE-FOR TABLE

dye	the skinny	where found	documented side effects
BLUE #1 (a.k.a. Brilliant Blue)	This food dye has been banned in France and Finland, but it's still widely used in the U.S.	• Baked goods • Candy • Cereal • Beverages	• Chromosomal damage in plant cells • Kidney tumors in mice • Asthma attacks
BLUE #2 (a.k.a. Indigo Carmine)	This could be the name of your toddler's hipster BFF, but it's illegal in Norway.	• Candy • Beverages • Dog food	• Brain tumors in male rats

TO-DYE-FOR TABLE (CONT.)

dye	the skinny	where found	documented side effects
GREEN #3 (a.k.a. Fast Green)	Banned in the European Union.	• Candy • Beverages • Ice cream • Cosmetics • Drugs	• Bladder tumors in male rats
RED #3 (a.k.a. Erythrosine)	In 1990, the FDA banned its use in cosmetics and topical drugs for causing tumors when applied externally, but it's still legal to use in food. Why?	• Baked goods • Candy • Sausages • Maraschino cherries	• Chromosomal damage in plant cells • Thyroid tumors in animals • Adverse effects in children's behavior
RED #40 (a.k.a. Allura Red)	Perhaps because of its alluring name, this is the most widely used and consumed artificial dye.	• Baked goods • Candy • Cereal • Beverages	• Chromosomal damage in plant cells • Lymphoma • Hyperactivity • Accelerated appearance of immune system tumors in mice • Allergy-like reactions in some individuals

dye	the skinny	where found	documented side effects
YELLOW #5 (a.k.a. Tartrazine)	A by-product of coal tar, this dye has been banned in Austria and Norway.	• Baked goods • Candy • Cereal • Beverages	• Chromosomal damage in plant cells • Asthma attacks • Lymphoma • Insomnia • Thyroid tumors • Allergy-like reactions • Aggression • Hyperactivity
YELLOW #6 (a.k.a. Sunset Yellow)	This may remind you of a beautiful California sunset, but it has been associated with many health concerns and has been banned in Norway and Sweden.	• Baked goods • Sausages • Cereal • Cosmetics • Beverages • Gelatin • Candy	• Chromosomal damage in plant cells • Asthma attacks • Eczema • Hives • Hyperactivity • Allergies • Adrenal tumors in animals

Green for Thought

Taking the toxic tables and other research into account, here are a few simple ideas to make your womb and home greener for you and your baby:

#1 *Opt for fresh food that is organic and free of dyes*

Before we get into it, I want to note that some organic crops are grown and processed with twenty-plus U.S. Organic Standard–approved synthetic substances such as ethanol, isopropanol, chlorine materials, copper sulfate, hydrogen peroxide, ozone gas, peracetic acid, petroleum-based plastic mulch, ammonium, etc. In order to find out what chemicals in what quantities were used in what crop, you'd have to call every rancher you or your grocery store buys from, which is obviously not realistic.

What's the point, then?

By opting for organic, you still avoid certain "badness," but, no: organic produce is not superhuman. The practical thing to do is to shop at your local farmers' market, wash your vegetables (organic or not), and eat them—because fresh food is really good for you! Now, on to why.

Why fresh, organic, and/or dye-free?

- The health benefits are blatant: You're avoiding preservatives, toxins, and additives that live in processed foods (canned or packaged). This is so important for your growing fetus.

- Growth hormones, antibiotics, and GMOs are prohibited or at least highly regulated in certified organic dairy and meats.

- Free-range, grass-fed, and grass-finished meat and dairy usually contains no antibiotics, with the animal raised under much healthier conditions, therefore producing more nutritious by-products.

- Products that eschew chemical dyes and instead use beets, carrots, spinach, pumpkin, berries, red cabbage, turmeric, saffron, and paprika to add color bring to the table (literally) all the health benefits that come with natural.

GMOS:
SUPERHEROES OR SUPERVILLAINS?

The jury is still out.

GMOs are Genetically Modified Organisms, created in laboratories by transferring DNA from one species to another in order to make crops stronger, bigger, tastier, and even more nutritious.

Sounds good, huh?

Well, these alien genes may come from viruses, insects, bacteria, and animals. Maybe even people.

Although GMOs' effects in humans haven't been sufficiently studied, foods that have been genetically modified are rumored to cause organ damage in lab animals and sterility in humans, and to trigger toxic and allergic reactions. Furthermore, some of the pollen stemming from genetically modified produce has been rumored to travel with the wind and land on milkweed, killing butterflies-to-be (caterpillars) that feed off them.

It makes you wonder what it could do to a fetus, right?

In addition to all this, introducing proteins to food increases the risk of new allergens, and altering food with antibiotic-resistant genes may increase their resistance in our population. (More on this issue in *Chapter 12: Sick Is a Four-Letter Word: Fussing Over a Fussy Baby.*)

The GMO debate is heated and just getting started. The science community has debunked many studies and it argues that there has never been a confirmed case of a negative health outcome in humans, animals, or the environment. Many former GMO-critics, including "The Science Guy" Bill Nye, have had a change of heart after delving further into the matter.

At the time of this writing, I still tend to favor organic foods (in which the USDA prohibits GMOs), but I no longer fear GMOs—at least for now. I'm keeping an open mind until further study is performed, reminding myself that a long time ago, some people believed the world was flat.

Good Foods That Help Flush Out Bad Toxins

Artichokes

Apples

Asparagus

Avocados

Basil

Beets

Blueberries

Brazil Nuts
(help expel mercury)

Broccoli

Cabbage

Cilantro
(helps expel mercury)

Cinnamon

Cranberries

Dandelion

Garlic

Ginger

Goji Berries

Grapefruit

Green Tea

Hemp

Kale

Lemon

Lemongrass

Onions

Pineapple

Seaweed
(helps expel heavy metals)

Turmeric

Watercress

Wheatgrass

#2 *Seek plant-based, all-natural skin-care products*

As with food, don't be afraid to read the ingredients in your baby's body wash. Skin is generally considered our largest organ, and dermal absorption is a sure way to expose you and your baby to toxic substances.

Why pay attention to ingredients you can't pronounce?

- Your body absorbs some of the chemicals you put on your skin; while pregnant or nursing, these could could cross the placental barrier or taint your breast milk.It goes without saying that your newborn's skin will also absorb anything you lather on her.

- Cosmetics, hair, and skincare products can contain harmful ingredients such as dioxane (a suspected carcinogenic) and phthalates.

- Aluminum is used in antiperspirants to block sweat glands, which some cite as a cause of breast cancer and memory problems. Although experts (including the National Cancer Institute and the Alzheimer's Association) agree there is no clear evidence of this, I used non-antiperspirant deodorant throughout my pregnancy and while breastfeeding. Besides, sweating is a way to rid your body of toxins, so why stop it? (My husband may have felt differently, but being the good guy he is, he never said anything about my BO.)

#3 *Favor plant-based and natural cleaning products*

Our home is like our family's amniotic sac, and as such we want to try to keep it as toxic-free as possible. I love disinfecting wipes as much as the next girl, but when at all possible I try to use natural cleaners such as vinegar and baking soda in my laundry, kitchen, bathroom, and specifically, my daughter's bedroom. Don't get me wrong: when there's shit and flus involved, I'm not shy with the Lysol. But I avoided it while pregnant and nursing, and I now use that type of stuff sparingly and as a last resort. I'm always surprised at how little elbow grease I need to scrub grime off my tub with baking soda.

Why not bleach?

- ⊕ The chemicals in your average household cleaner have harmful toxins that pollute your environment, eventually making it into your baby's hands, mouth, and lungs.

- ⊕ Use of chemical products pollutes the water supply in our communities, which makes it back into our parks and homes.

BIG NO-NO!

Keep Away from Little Hands

Most household cleaners contain chlorine, triclosan, 2-butoxyethanol, and quaternary ammonium compounds (a.k.a. quats). They can be deadly if ingested.

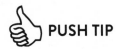 **PUSH TIP**

Keep the poison control number on speed dial and remember to share with caregivers. The American Association of Poison Control Centers 24-hour hotline is (800) 222-1222.

#4 *Install a water filter or reverse-osmosis filtration system, or use a pitcher with a built-in carbon filter*

It took me a bit to get around to this one, but at some point I had to stop buying water by the case. We currently use a good ol' Brita for ourselves (which doesn't really remove fluoride) and buy spring water by the gallon for our daughter. Next step: Install a fancy water filtration system in our home.

Why avoid tap?

- ⊕ Tap water may contain traces of contaminants such as chlorine, lead, and arsenic.

- ⊕ Tap water is fortified with fluoride, which in recent years has become controversial.

THE FLUORIDE IN TAP WATER DEBATE

**by Heather Juergensen,
Founder of TheStrongWoman.net, Los Angeles, CA,
Mother of Two**

Many intelligent people are asking "Why?" to the question of fluoride in drinking water. I could see that if we and our children had very few cavities, it would be a no-brainer to leave fluoride in the water. But that's not what has happened.

You'll find thousands of articles on either side and it is incredibly hard to cut through the noise and see what's actually true. I am personally always intrigued when someone who has sat firmly on one side of an argument eventually comes out on the other side.

Richard and Karilee Shames, a doctor-nurse team whose specialty is thyroid health, were for years conventionally pro-fluoridation. After reading hundreds of articles and books, they changed their minds, due to serious concerns about the particular fluoride we put in our water being a potential hormone disruptor. "We learned that the source of fluoride for municipalities is not sodium fluoride, the compound used by researchers to determine benefit versus risk," they noted. "Instead...we found that what is added to almost all city water when it is fluoridated is the industrial waste product hydrofluosilicic acid."

I'm not a fanatic on this issue, but it fascinates me that plenty of evidence shows genuine risk to having this fluoride in our drinking water, while little evidence exists that it is preventing cavities.

So, as a society, why are we leaving it in our drinking water?

#5 *Consider cloth diapers, hybrids, or eco-friendly, chlorine-free disposable diapers*

My road to hell was paved with green intentions. My name's Ivette and I'm a disposable diaper addict. I know they take about five hundred years to decompose and that manufacturing them cost us more resources than the saintly cloth diaper, but I can't help it: They make my life so much easier. Imagine what our great-grandmothers would've accomplished had they been able to use disposable diapers!

That's why I find eco-friendly disposable diapers such a good compromise. However, they tend to be pricey and sometimes not well-crafted.

Like all the choices in motherhood, this one is yours. But here are some perks if you follow the green brick road:

Why cloth, hybrids, or eco-friendly disposables?

- 🌐 Unlike most disposable diapers, cloth and hybrid diapers are free of harmful chemicals.

- 🌐 Most eco-friendly disposable diapers are made with no chemicals, or very few compared to their counterparts.

- 🌐 Using cloth or hybrids reduces landfill waste.

- 🌐 Eco-friendly diapers disintegrate faster than regular ones.

- 🌐 Washing your cloth diapers and/or hybrid shells at home saves money (estimated cost = $20/month vs. $60/month for disposables).

For Further Viewing

Cloth diapers have come a long way since the old days and using them is way easier than it used to be. If you're considering this option, look up this awesome video called **"Types of Cloth Diapers (and How to Use Them)"** by Plus1Please on YouTube. It'll tell you everything you need to know!

#6 *Use glass bottles and containers*

I was scared of glass baby bottles at first, because I thought they would be breakable and therefore dangerous. Turns out, they're pretty durable.

Why glass?

- Unlike plastic, no toxins can leach from glass into consumable liquids or foods.

- Glass has a longer shelf life and can be recycled over and over back into its glass form.

Sustaining a Green Mindset for the Next Generation

Being green is not just about putting stuff in the recycling can. In fact, I recently found out that they won't recycle a lot of what I put in the blue bin. I was heartbroken to find out my old socks aren't being reincarnated.

I've also learned that being green means I have to promote sustainability. We hear this word tossed about in every menu around the hip block, and it can be confusing to pin down the exact definition.

But if you know how healthy relationships work, then you understand sustainability. It's balancing your give-and-take. A symbiosis. I scratch your back and you scratch mine. Simply, if we take care of our planet, it will take care of us.

Everything that we need for our survival and well-being is dependent on our native resources (land, food, water, etc.). Our planet will be our children's children's planet, and our actions now will greatly impact its state by that time. The goal of sustainability is to develop and maintain a system by which humans and nature can coexist indefinitely, thus ensuring enough resources for future generations. Sustainability is all about practicing good karma with Mother Earth.

In my home, I take small strides towards sustainability by being frugal with what I buy, use, and eat, taking only what I need. I also try to avoid products that are bad for our planet, and us, by default. When my daughter grows up, I hope to impart this responsibility to her so that she can help her generation keep this world alive for five billion years more.

Sometimes being green isn't practical or affordable. Every day, I have to make small choices with big repercussions—either sacrifice my own sanity or do right by the planet. I can't say the planet always wins.

Step by Step

Even if we deserted our chemical-ridden, diaper-infested homes and moved off the grid to live off the land, we would encounter harmful shit. Not to mention hungry bears. So don't let all these facts and ideas bring anxiety to your life. Stress is toxic to your body, too!

We've come a long way from drinking water out of a hose, getting mercury fillings, and eating Spam out of a can. We've learned that in order to avoid toxins, we need to recognize them and understand their potential harm. Armed with our newfound knowledge, we can do a risk/benefit assessment on a case-by-case basis. Putting your baby in a pair of flame-retardant PJs is probably not going to stunt her development, but if you know it can be harmful, you may choose differently next time you shop. And maybe manufacturers will look at their loss reports and stop using such products in their merchandise. We can all be a small link in the chain of change.

Tackle as much or as little as your lifestyle allows. Even getting a few small plants to spruce up the place may help reduce airborne chemicals in your home. It's all about those baby steps.

Here's a nifty page summing up all the culprits. Snap a picture of it or simply tear out the page and stick it on your fridge for easy reference.

RECOMMENDED DAILY SUPPLEMENT INTAKE FOR PREGNANCY

Folate	400–600 mgs
Omega 3/DHA	300 mgs
Protein	75–100 grams
Calcium	1,000 mgs
Magnesium	350–360 mgs
Iron	27–44 mgs
Vitamin D	600–4,000 IU
B6	1.9 mgs
B12	2.6 mcg

BFFS
(BEST FRIENDS FOREVER)

Calcium + Vitamin D
Calcium + Magnesium
Iron + Vitamin C

BFS
(BITTER FOES)

Calcium + Iron

SHOPPING LIST
(CIRCLE OR HIGHLIGHT)

Avocados
Bananas
Strawberries
Blueberries
Raspberries
Blackberries
Oranges
Figs
Apricots
(dried or fresh)
Raisins
Oatmeal
Beans
Chickpeas
(or hummus)

Lentils
Quinoa
Edamame
Almonds
Brazilian Nuts
Nut Butters
(all-natural)
Hazelnuts
Pumpkin Seeds
Sunflower Seeds
Chia Seeds
Papaya
Spinach
Kale
Okra

Asparagus
Artichokes
Brussel Sprouts
Broccoli
Green Beans
Cauliflower
Sweet Potatoes
Beef (grass-fed)
Poultry
(pasture-raised)
Pork
Oysters
Salmon
(wild-caught,
Alaskan or sockeye)

Haddock
Shrimp
Sardines
Catfish
Mackerel
Scallops
Seaweed
Dairy (grass-fed)
Yogurt
Cheese
Eggs (free-range)
Whole Grains
Olive Oil
(cold-pressed)

HEALTHY SNACK FAVES

BAD PLASTICS

3   6   7

OKAY PLASTICS

1   2   4   5

VILLAIN DYES

Blue #1   (Brilliant Blue)
Blue #2   (Indigo Carmine)
Green #3   (Fast Green)
Red #3   (Erythrosine)
Red #40   (Allura Red)
Yellow #5   (Tartrazine)
Yellow #6   (Sunset Yellow)

THIS MEANS PHTHALATES

DBP
DEP
DEHP
BIs
BzBP
DMP

BUY ORGANIC

Alfalfa
Apples
Beef
Blueberries (domestic)
Celery
Corn
Formula
Grapes
Hawaiian Papaya
Kale and Collard Greens
Lettuce
Milk
Nectarines
Peaches
Potatoes
Soy By-products
Spinach
Strawberries
Sugar Beets
Sweet Bell Peppers
Sweetened Juices
Tomatoes
Yellow Squash
Zucchini

THIS MEANS PFCS

Fluoro
Perfluoro

SKIP ORGANIC LABELS

Asparagus
Avocados
Broccoli
Cabbage
Cantaloupe
Carrots
Cauliflower
Eggplant
Grapefruit
Honeydew
Kiwi
Mango
Mushrooms
Onions
Pineapple
Sweet Peas
Watermelon

7 SERIOUSLY.

How Much Crap Does a Teeny-Weeny Little Baby Need?

YOU PERUSE THE INTERNET, trying not to eat the entire pint of Sir Dazs...thanking the smart folk who made it possible for you to shop from home in your holed pajamas. Can you imagine having to *walk* through a store and actually *talk* to people in order to determine what, which brand, and how many of each item to put on your registry? Without consulting consumer reviews or ratings? Or price-checking?!

Most of all, you wonder how moms in third world villages survive without any of this shit.

I mean, selecting the right stroller is comparable to taking a starving child through Baskin Robbins' 31 Flavors. The choices and combinations are inexhaustible. There's a stroller that can charge your phone and track the miles you've walked. That's impressive, but I'm holding out for one with a changing table and built-in bidet that can fold inside my purse. Stroller gods be damned, I could use a constant source of freshness down there.

Speaking of which, the butt-wipe market has gone all sorts of niche. They make wipes for every single orifice your baby has. Actually, they haven't tapped into belly button real estate yet, but the boogie wipes are a bestseller and I'm amongst their most loyal consumers. The saline pulls the boogers OUT!

Boogie wipes aside, I'm a minimalist. I am constantly purging stuff from my house to keep up with my collector-husband packing in more. When I die, I don't want to subject my grieving family to sorting through piles of knickknacks just because I didn't have the courage to part with them. It's not like I'm King Tut and I'm gonna need all this crap in my crypt, yo!

So when I made my baby list, I tried to keep the paraphernalia to a minimum. We didn't want to be surrounded by colorful plastic shit that sings hard-to-forget tunes every time you bump into it or have to hunt down a magnet every time we wanted to use a knife. Visitors always remark on how little evidence they see of a toddler living in our house. However, in order to achieve this, we've sacrificed the ability to relax. Every room in our home contains a booby trap for our child. Our daughter's bedroom is the only safe place she can roam free, as unsupervised as a toddler can be. I know this is unsustainable for saner parents—but hey, this is the road we chose to waddle.

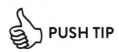 **PUSH TIP**

Thrifty Mama

Before leaving the hospital, grab as many goodies as they're willing to give. We made out like bandits, walking out with a wheelchair-load of diapers, wipes, burp cloths, shirts, hats, a brush, a thermometer, a plastic bin to hold it all...plus, a perfectly good, brand new baby!!!.

You may choose a more reasonable path and build a toy heaven inside a gated area that safely barricades your child. This will give you the freedom to enjoy a warm cup of coffee or even run into the next room for a quickie. Or maybe your octomom ass is expecting eight babies, and a surplus of bright-colored distractions will be the only thing between you and an asylum. *Or,* maybe you live in a castle with uniformed maids and have an extra wing just for Baby.

Whatever your situation, you're entitled to choose what, which, and how many your baby gets. Fortunately—and especially if this is your first baby—you get the luxury of making a registry so people can help you stock up.

Baby List & Registry

Your baby list contains everything you need and want for your bun-in-the-oven. This "master list" will be a drawing board for your registry. Your registry specifies desired items that others can gift to you to help you get locked and loaded.

I learned the concept of these two lists the hard way: My own registry included *everything* I might possibly want, and I ended up receiving a lot of "optional" items at my shower and not enough "must have's." I recommend putting only priority and gift-suitable items on your public registry. Remember: The Internet doesn't run out of shit. Ever. You don't need to have everything all at once. But also keep in mind that you have only one chance to score a bounty of free baby gear.

The pressure is on—and not just your pelvis.

Baby Registry Confidential

Before you set out to create your baby list and registry, here are a few points to consider.

#1 *Be practical*

Don't get stuff that's going to make your life harder or that won't fit in your home. Consider the storage in your closets and kitchen as well as the amenities you already have at your disposal.

For example, do you have a dishwasher? Then get as many kitchen items as you can get dirty. Since we don't, I never got a baby blender because the thought of having to wash it made me want to purée my own pruned fingers.

Being practical and simplifying routines will make it easier to care for your baby (and you).

#2 *Keep it real, yo!*

The definition of "realistic," according to my computer's dictionary, is: *having or showing a sensible and practical idea of what can be achieved or expected.* So, beyond objective practicality, know yourself and your limitations. Embrace them, even. It's what makes you *you*.

Easier said than done, I know. I'm one to talk. I often let my decisions be clouded by the version of myself I want to be rather than who I really am. And that can lead to clutter real fast.

To further explore the "practical" example from above, owning a little food processor, for me, would've been not only impractical but unrealistic. I wouldn't have used it. I simply don't have the required dedication to make organic chicken soup from scratch, blend it, package it, and freeze it. If you do (and have a dishwasher), get that food maker stat. Feel free to make extra and share with a mom like me, who wishes I were more into cooking from scratch than I am.

It's hard to foresee what you'll really need or what will work for your family until your baby is born. But being honest about your

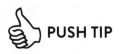 **PUSH TIP**

The "Triple-R" Rule: Return, Resell, or Re-gift

Despite your best efforts to register for things you will use, it may turn out you don't—and aren't going to. Or you get duplicate gifts or want more recent, upgraded versions of items. For this reason, keep all boxes and receipts so you can return unused (or barely used) items, resell, or re-gift.

My family knows I'm a pretty unabashed re-gifter. My motto is: *Somebody's trash...*

110

lifestyle may keep you from beating yourself up for not ever using that jogger stroller. Because if you were never a runner before you got pregnant, chances are, pushing a baby out of your vajayjay isn't magically going to turn you into one. And even for someone who is used to running, it can be tough after delivery. I tried it and with every bounce, I had gunk gushing out from between my legs (in addition to milk sprinklers on my nipples). I was a wet hot mess that American summer.

#3 *Be true to your inner mama*

Embrace your inner self and aim to acquire whatever rocks your boat. Be it traditional or abstract; gender-oriented or neutral; U.S.A.-made or child-labored (well, maybe not this)—it's your shower, your baby, and you're the one pushing. Compiling your registry should be a fun and unique experience. Strive to make all the items reflect you and your partner.

I'm all about practicality, so I went with the eyesore generic diaper backpack instead of the designer-made bag; the baby sling that gifts a second sling to a mom in a third world country (I never used it—I hope she did); and splurged on a vintage doctor's baby examination table. I felt really good about those choices because they reflected who I am as a person and my own style.

#4 *Be considerate to the mother of all mothers*

When buying a new product, you can set out to find recyclable, sustainable, and/or recycled products. And if you're really into being green—or simply wanna save money—this is a perfectly valid question to voice out loud when making your baby list: *Can I find it used?*

Most large baby items such as activity centers, play yards, strollers, and bathtubs are quickly outgrown, therefore relatively easy to acquire nearly new. Furniture, such as cribs, changing stations, dressers, etc., are other big-ticket items that usually hold up over time. You can procure previously loved items via family, mom groups, Craigslist, consignment stores, and social media.

Last but not least, cloth diapers and hybrid diapers are very popular these days. I highly endorse them, as does Mother Earth. But don't buy them if Planet Mom can't sustain the process. Returning to the previous guidelines, you gotta find the most practical and realistic shit-collecting method that's true to your inner self.

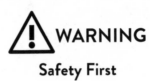

WARNING

Safety First

It is very important that when buying anything, especially used, you research the product and read all safety instructions for it. You want to make sure there haven't been any recalls, durability restrictions, safety concerns, or anything that could jeopardize your baby's well-being. Additionally, be wary of procuring secondhand humidifiers, mattresses, linens, or anything with absorbent materials. Babies and breastfeeding mamas excrete many fluids that can seep into the threads and become host to a mold and bacteria party. However, this doesn't include apparel as that's easy to disinfect. Babies go through clothes so fast that hand-me-downs and thrift-wear is way vintage cool.

#5 *Choose your own registry adventure*

A wealth of physical and online stores offer registry services. Several of my friends set up registries with multiple stores and that worked out well for them and their guests. Also, chains like Target and Babies"R"Us offer perks for registering with them, such as bonus gift cards and discounts. And these stores are typically easier for the older crowd; Aunt Jo's idea of "browsing" may be to go window-shopping at the local mall wearing her Sunday best.

Most of our relatives and friends are pretty Internet-savvy, so we decided to use the website babyli.st (Baby List Baby Registry). This website allows you to list items from a variety of online outlets. My Registry and Amazon also offer "universal" registries. Amazon's is kind of unsightly but very practical. Baby List, while super cute, made our guests mark items as "reserved" and then come back to update the registry once the item was purchased. I got a few duplicate gifts because of this (though that did provide some great items for my re-gift bin).

It's fun to compile a list of things for baby. It's sweet to imagine her in snuggly clothes, holding a lovey in her carefully curated nursery. Enjoy the process of selecting all the props. Registries are such a great look into a mom's mind. I love examining a registry and guessing what kind of mom put it together: Is she practical, traditional, stylish, eco-conscious...?

What's your style?

Once you determine what you need based on your style and lifestyle, take a gander at your registry options. Consider what may be convenient for you, your hosts, and your guests. Then register and don't stress...nothing is set in stone. You can keep editing your registry even after baby is born, and can return things you decide you don't want or need.

List o' Crap and Goodies You May (or May Not) Need

Figuring out what all to buy and put on the registry really overwhelmed me. I spent a lot of time perusing reviews, forums, boards, and blogs, asking friends, trying things, returning things, and never using things in order to become an "expert." You'll be a whiz soon enough, too.

To assist you on the DIY registry road, I've put together a list of baby items, with the insights I gained about each. Some you'll want to get yourself, some you'll want to put on your registry, and some you'll decide you don't need at all. Keep in mind that what worked for me may not work for you. So take out your red pen and check off the things you think you'll use!

Please note that nobody paid me to place their products on this list or to review them—these are my true and honest opinions.

ITEM, THE SKINNY, AND THEN SOME MORE

FOR NURSERY

❑ **Crib**

The place your baby sleeps. Or not. If you're planning on co-sleeping or using a bassinet in your room, there's no need for a crib. If space allows and you want one, acquire a convertible one that will transform into a toddler bed.

❑ **Crib Mattress**

If you get a crib, you'll need a mattress. Most crib mattresses come with a soft side and a firmer side to reduce the risk of Sudden Infant Death Syndrome (SIDS) when your baby is a newborn. Once your baby turns one, you can flip to the softer side.

Beyond that, choices can be overwhelming.

One conundrum can be whether to go synthetic or organic. "Synthetic bedding products may expose you to longer term concerns of airborne plastics, VOCs, carcinogens, and flame retardants," says Silver Lake mom Eve, "[while] natural bedding products are less successful at counteracting the dust mites and other microbes that aggravate allergies." Experts recommend bedding made from nonsynthetic materials such as cotton, wool, silk, bamboo, hemp, and/or plastic materials made from food-grade polyethylene.

We decided on a Serta organic crib mattress for our daughter. Naturepedic also has great reviews. Regardless of brand, this is not the time to skimp. Babies sleep 50 to 60 percent of their day, so they deserve a good, clean, safe place to lay their little bodies.

❏ **Crib Sheet**

A fitted sheet that covers the mattress. You'll probably get a few of these regardless, so maybe leave them off the registry. I got so many that I ended up re-gifting a few. *Shhh!*

❏ **Crib Mattress Pad**

A fitted protective cover that goes between the crib sheet and the mattress. Buy one and put another on the registry so you'll have two. That way, you won't have to hurry up and wash the soiled one in the middle of the night. And make sure you get one that is water resistant. Otherwise, the accident will leak right through to the mattress.

❏ **Crib Bumper Pad**

A cushioned wraparound liner for the inside of your crib. Bumpers are mainly decorative, though they do protect baby's limbs from being jammed between the crib slats and cushion his head from hitting against them. However, the American Academy of Pediatrics (AAP) recommends against them entirely, for risk of SIDS or suffocation.

I know plenty of mothers who have used bulky, padded ones to no harm, but I favor the thin kind made with breathable fabrics. In the end, I opted out of this completely because I'm still wary and also, I don't like to add more things to my laundry list. Literally.

❑ **Bassinet or Bedside Sleeper**

A place you can set baby to sleep safely. As a minimalist, I recommend getting one only if it's the sleep furniture you're planning on using for the first months of your baby's life and/or you're planning on sharing Z's. They even make special bassinets that connect to your bed, called a co-sleeper or beside sleeper.

You may also want to invest in a bassinet if you need a second place to put your baby to sleep. Getting one on wheels is convenient, as you can move it easily from room to room while your baby snoozes. Bassinets also come as part of travel stroller systems and it can be practical to get one you can snap onto your stroller legs.

❑ **Glider or Rocking Chair**

A rocking chair or glider will come in handy to cozily feed your baby and/or rock him to sleep. We used to bounce ours on a yoga ball instead, which was great for my ass and the only thing that made her stop crying. However, unless you're gymnast, a ball is not ideal for nursing.

❑ **Changing Table**

This is where you change your baby. Get one only if the storage/shelving beneath it is worth it to you. If not, you'll be left with a piece of furniture you can't easily repurpose.

❑ **Changing Pad**

The concave mattress you affix to a changing table—or any another flat surface, such as a dresser—to change baby's diaper on. I recommend getting something you can hose off.

❑ **Changing Pad Cover**

The fitted sheet that goes over the changing pad. I recommend you get at least two, maybe more. You'll be washing it (and shit off of it) a lot.

❑ **Hamper**

This is where your baby's unmentionables go until you wash them. Unless you're sharing a room with your child, get the nursery its own hamper. When your child gets older, he'll learn to put clothes there himself.

❑ **Mobile**

A soothing decorative structure you suspend from the crib or ceiling for baby to look up at. This is completely a matter of preference. We chose to go without the extra stimulus.

You can make your own mobile if you're into DIY stuff or Etsy has pretty cool ones, too.

❑ **Sound Machine**

An appliance that provides soundscapes for optimal sleeping and relaxation. I'm all about white noise, but the soothing sound of a fan or air purifier works just as well.

❑ **Nightlight or Lamp**

A registry staple, unless you have dimmers for your lights.

PEE & POO PARAPHERNALIA

❑ **Diapers**

Diapers are a much-needed commodity for new parents and, hence, a great thing to register for, as it's a recurring expense. It can be tough to choose between disposables (just choosing a brand is challenging enough), cloth, and hybrids. In *Chapter 6: My Green Alter-Mama: Baby Steps Toward a Healthier Home and Womb*, we discussed the benefits of choosing green diapers and concluded that you gotta pick the most practical shit-catching solution for your lifestyle.

Other than going al fresco, here are your options:

❑ **Disposable Diapers**

Easy peasy, lemon squeezy...disposable diapers make it all breezy. The con? Well, it's a lot of waste. However, brands such as Honest and Seventh Generation make diapers with less harmful chemicals that may take slightly less time to decompose. Broody Chick diapers are fully compostable; however, based on consumer reviews, it seems they may still need perfecting in terms of functionality.

❑ **Cloth Diapers**

Companies such as Blessed Bums periodically pick up your soiled diapers and supply you with fresh ones. They take care of all the washing. My Great-Grandma Mamita would've killed a few chickens with her bare hands for that service.

❑ **Hybrid Diapers**

The great compromise: The main shell is a waterproof cloth cover that you can reuse. In it, you insert a disposable liner that you can throw out instead of washing.

These come in a variety of colors, sizes, and brands. Those who use them advise testing out a few to find the one that best fits your baby's bottom. Also, you can buy used shells—I often see them posted in my online mom forum groups.

❑ **Disposable Baby Wipes**

Moist towelettes to clean your baby's privates during every diaper change. For the first couple of months, you may want to use wet gauze pads or flannel wipes. I also really liked Water Wipes, which are 99.9 percent water. Afterwards, I tried Earth's Best (too dry), Huggies Naturals (broke apart too easily), and finally settled for Babyganics (felt just right!).

❑ **Flannel Wipes**

Reusable cloth wipes made out of soft natural fibers. Moisten them with water to wipe butts, faces, and runny noses. Then throw them in the wash to reuse over and over again.

❑ **Baby Wipe Dispenser**

A container that keeps your baby wipes moist and helps dispense them as needed. These are practical. It's nice to not have to peel back plastic tape every time you need to get into your wipes.

❑ **Baby Wipe Warmer**

A container that keeps your baby wipes warm. For practical reasons, I try to avoid unnecessary electrical appliances in my baby's room. Plus, my one friend who swears by the warmer admitted that her baby got upset if ever she encountered a cold wipe. The image of my daughter throwing a temper tantrum in a public restroom over a cold wipe on her butt was all I needed to decide we were sticking with room temperature.

❑ **Diaper Pail**

A trashcan designed specifically for diapers.

I feel pretty strongly about using pails with a *sliding* door. I also recommend a receptacle that can be used with any regular trash bag or laundry bag.

I despise cans with doors that push downward. Those things deserve to be full of shit. You can't fit as many dirty diapers because you need room for the lid to go down, and when your trash starts to get full—and the can is tiny—your hand is forced to touch the diapers piled up inside. To boot, most of that type don't take regular bags, so you have to open the unit and pull out the specially designed bag (which looks like sausage casing) from underneath, cut it, and tie it.

All of this is just too much shit-handling for my taste.

Advocates claim that this design contains odors better. Maybe that's true, but I'm not sure I'm ready for the Pepsi challenge.

❑ **Disposable Diaper Bags**
I call these human poop bags. They're individual trash bags for your diapers. Since I try to avoid plastic, I compromised by using biodegradable dog poop bags for this purpose. They're absolutely handy when on the go, also to transport soiled clothing (a.k.a. hazardous waste) back home. Some people also bag poopy diapers at home to avoid smelly bins. Alternatively, I sometimes flush number twos down the toilet and then toss out the diaper.

❑ **Diaper Sprayer**
If you commit to cloth diapers, your life will be much easier if you get this hose that attaches to the toilet. It's used to rinse the soiled cloth diaper after you dump the poop in the bowl. Then you can throw the wet, (hopefully)

residue-free cloth or reusable liner into your hamper. Wash wet linens within two days to avoid mold growth.

❑ **Pee-Pee Teepee**

A felt cone you put over your baby's penis to prevent him from giving you a golden shower. I have a daughter, so I asked a supermom of two boys. Her assessment: "It just seems like one more small item to keep up with that would never be in the right place at the right time. I either take my chances or cover old faithful with a diaper." She's a wise mama.

BREASTFEEDING BOUNTY

❑ **Nursing/Feeding Pillow**

A U-shaped pillow you set around your waist to bolster your baby for a more comfortable feeding position (bottle or breast). It's also great for propping your kid in different positions through different stages. I really liked my Boppy pillow, but Ergobaby also has one that looks amazing.

❑ **Nursing Bras & Clothes**

Clothing specifically designed for easy access to your breasts. Most of them clip open and shut so you can pop out that nipple with the snap of your fingers.

You're probably on your own with this. Nobody wants to buy you a nursing bra except maybe your mom or your Aunt Jo who burned her own bra in the sixties.

My favorite nursing bras are Basics brand from Target; I bought fancy ones and never used them. I have two friends who also swear by Basics and regret purchasing anything else.

I'm also all about getting any kind of underwear brand new. Based on the well-worn condition of my own nursing bras, I wouldn't want to buy anybody else's crusty old brassiere. Especially if I don't know where that boob's been!

❏ **Breastfeeding Accessories**

Items such as nipple cream and nursing pads. I think these are better left on your private baby list—do you really want to model breast pads at your shower?

For me, the Nuk Ultra Thin Nursing Pads were the absolute best. The others felt like wearing an overnight pad versus a panty liner. The downside? If you overflow, you may be sporting wet rings on your shirt. But I found them absorbent enough and I didn't want the extra "padding" as I was already rocking a Pam Anderson breastfeeding rack.

If you've got green intentions, you can buy washable breast pads. They're super soft and come in a variety of colors, patterns, and shapes. Now that I'm done breastfeeding, I use mine as face cleansing pads.

❏ **Breast Pump**

A device that attaches to your nipple and sucks breast milk into a container.

❏ **Electric Breast Pump**

If you're planning on breastfeeding, bite the nipple and acquire this barbaric invention. But before you purchase or put it on the registry, check with your insurance carrier, as some might shoulder the cost or help finance it.

I also think buying used is safe as long as you replace all the piping. Also, if you're planning on PWD (Pump While Driving), consider getting an AC car adapter so you can plug in during your commute and pump with reckless abandon. PWD is still technically legal in all fifty states, though you may be issued a warning. For safety reasons, it may be a good idea to pull over to "connect" and "disconnect."

❑ **Manual Breast Pump**
A manual breast pump is cheap, and a great way to collect mother's milk while on the go.

❑ **Breast Milk Storage Bags and Containers**
These niftily attach to your pump gear to collect the nectar of the moms, which you can then store inside the fridge or freezer, depending on when you think you'll need the milk. The best type of receptacle is one you can turn into a bottle fast, be it a pouch you click onto a bottle or a container with a nipple attachment. Most pump brands have a line of compatible milk-collecting and feeding gear.

❑ **Bustier Pumping Bra**
A specially designed brassiere that attaches to a pump's suction cups so you can move around freely while you pump. I think this is a must if you need to pump a lot; otherwise, you have to sit like a dunce in the corner of the room, holding those suction cups in place.

FEEDING STUFF

❑ **Bottles**
Most babies are particular about their bottles. Register for a small sampling of bottles and nipples and then invest in the lot once your baby chooses.

Glass is the new black and most durable, but most moms choose plastic. Plastic bottles don't hold up as well, but you can donate used ones to animal shelters when done. If using hand-me-down glass bottles, replace old nipples with brand new ones.

❑ **Bottle Brush**

A brush with a long handle perfect for getting to the bottom of things. Bottles do need washing.

❑ **Formula**

A source of nourishment for your infant that you can use on its own or in tandem with breast milk. Most formulas can be used until your baby is a year old. After that, you can move to milk or toddler formula if desired. Watch out for sugar and additives, though. For more details, check out "Ingredients To Consider Avoiding When Buying Formula" in *Chapter 13: Breastfeeding Sucks: Pumping's Just Another Word for Nothing Left to Lose.*

If you're planning to formula-feed your baby, you may want to buy in bulk, but only after you find a formula that works. Do your research and try your preferred brand out of the gate, but know that your baby may have sensitivities, so it may take you a bit to find the perfect fit (lactose-free, goat's milk, soy-based, etc.).

Lots of moms sell unopened formulas online. Buying from them can save you some moola!

❑ **Formula Dispenser**

It's a Keurig for formula!

These machines are pricey but, although not a necessity, they can help keep Mama sane. Lovers of this product claim that it keeps bottle-making consistent;

formula is always brewed precisely and to the perfect temperature, no matter who makes it—or, rather, presses the button. It's a great tool for a busy parent. The most high-tech ones even automatically order the formula pods for you when you're running low!

It's important to note that some of these machines are brand-affiliated and only usable with their particular formula "pods." If this is the toy for you, find one that is compatible with most major brands or if you're already partial to a specific brand of formula, find the machine that supports your brand's "pods."

❑ **Bottle Drying Rack**

A special wooden, metal, or plastic rack to dry your baby's stuff. When I gave birth, everyone had the Boon Grass Countertop rack and I bought into it. I didn't like it because the "grass" got nasty underneath, making it one more thing I had to scrub. If you have limited counter space, a regular drying rack, and/or are planning on breastfeeding a lot, a special rack is not worth it. But if you're pumping and/or using formula, you may find one useful.

❑ **Dishwasher Basket**

A basket to keep your baby's little items from spinning through the dishwasher. This can provide a good safety net for some of your gear; if breast pump flanges get tossed around during a wash cycle they can very well go "swimming with the fishes."

Silicone or BPA- and phthalate-free plastics are best for high temperatures.

❑ **Sterilizing Steam Bags**

Bags you heat in the microwave with water to sterilize bottles, pacifiers, and pump gear. In my opinion, a good bath in boiling water does the trick. Also, these seemed like a safety hazard for a klutzy mom like me. However, these could be useful if traveling or while pumping at the office.

If you're green-minded and/or want to save a little money, hunt for reusable sterilization steam bags such as EnviroPouch.

❑ **High Chair, Hook-On Chair, or Booster Seat**

Options to seat your child safely while she eats. Most high chairs (unless you can afford Stokke stuff) are eyesores and a PIA to clean. Hook-on chairs are foldable and easily portable, and they clamp on to most tables. Weight restrictions vary, but the Lobster Chair handles up to forty-five pounds of baby. Booster seats fasten to most chairs and usually grow with your kid.

After two recommendations, we went for the super-affordable Fisher-Price Healthy Care Deluxe Booster Seat, which also works for toddlers and is easy to wipe clean. I've even hosed it down on a few extra-messy occasions. Yeah, plastic does have a few practical perks.

❑ **Baby Food Maker**

There's an entire market of these baby blenders...which basically do the same thing as a regular blender, but on a smaller scale. If you don't have a blender, maybe invest in something the entire family can use, since babies only eat puréed food for so long. Or find an all-in-one model that purées AND steams your food. These are reasonably priced and can still be useful after baby outgrows purées. Because once they master that pincer grip and fall for finger food, they may resist being spoon-fed.

It's very hip these days to practice baby-led weaning (letting your child feed herself safe finger foods from the get-go), which means no more glop. However, I recently read something that made sense to me: Purées help ensure your baby gets more nutrients per bite. Food for thought, ladies.

❑ **Reusable Baby Food Containers**
Receptacles for storing food in the fridge and/or freezer and transporting to-go snacks. Definitively a must.

❑ **Table-Ready: Bowls, Spoons, Sippy Cups, Bibs, Splat Mat**
There's a whole wide world out there made out of stainless steel, rubber, maple wood, recycled milk jugs— you name it. You won't need this stuff for a while and something better may hit the stands by the time you do, so I wouldn't register for it. Also, you don't know if your baby will prefer a straw or a sippy cup. And for solids, we used the high chair tray for a long time before graduating to bowls and plates. You want the food to be the only thing your baby can fling across the room.

GADGETS THAT COULD CONTAIN YOUR BABY WHILE YOU GO NÚMERO 2:

❑ **Portable Crib**
A portable crib provides a safe place for your baby to sleep or play. It's a great big-ticket item to list on your registry.

If you travel a lot, this is a must and there are many lightweight options on the market. A portable crib can also conveniently allow your baby to sleep in your room. If your baby is crawling but not cruising yet, a crib that doubles as a small, cushioned playpen can keep him safely contained while you do whatever you need to do. If he's cruising (walking supported and along the edges of furniture), it's not advisable to leave him in there unsupervised, as he may be able to knock the entire thing onto its side.

Another downside to all this: Despite the varied designs available, they're all eyesores.

❑ **Play Yard**

These are fairly portable gates that can safely contain your child. But the same cruising advice for portable cribs goes for this. Other than that, as long as it's properly built, the props within the walls are child-safe and the floor is padded, so you can take a pretty big dump while your baby hangs out in the playpen. But never be out of earshot. In fact, rig up the camera and bring the video monitor inside the bathroom.

Buy a play yard that you can also safely use outdoors. It can be great at a campsite, the beach, or any other environment that would normally require not only your full attention, but your full body, on alert. This way, you can stow your child within the portable walls, place your chair outside Baby Town, and sip a drink while looking out at the ocean—until your baby decides she'd rather be in your arms, that is.

❏ Infant Glider, Rocker, or Swing

A portable seat that soothes your baby by rocking, swinging, or gliding her. I recommend getting something that can grow with your child instead of becoming obsolete.

My husband was sold on the Mamaroo, which offers a variety of computerized movements and sounds. However, it's super-expensive and only good for about six months; once baby is strong enough to sit up, she will lean forward and can tip the entire thing down with her.

I wish I would've bought the Nuna Leaf Bouncer instead, which converts into a chair for later use. The Rock 'n Play and the Papasan are also popular brands in this rockin' realm.

BIG NØ-NØ!

Avoid SIDS and Positional Asphyxia

Rockers, swings, or gliders are not recommended for sleep. The same advisory goes for car seats.

Sleeping in a non-flat position increases risk of SIDS and positional asphyxia (when the air flow to baby's head is cut off by being slumped forward while sleeping). This position may block airways or prevent the chest from fully expanding, causing suffocation.

❑ **Bouncer Seat or Exersaucer**

A device designed to stimulate your baby's physical and motor growth while providing a safe space to leave her while you go make coffee. These were invaluable for a lot of my mom friends, but we bought our Jumparoo a bit late in the game (she was ten months), so our daughter used it maybe ten times.

❑ **Bumbo Seat**

A portable chair for your baby, which can be great for feeding. Despite some warnings about postural effects (see text box), we still gave the Bumbo a try, as many people think they're fine if not used for prolonged periods of time. Unfortunately, our daughter's thighs were too fat to fit through the leg holes!

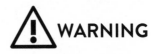 **WARNING**

Stick 'Em Straight

Mary Weck, clinical coordinator of Physical Therapy at Children's Memorial Hospital in Chicago, was quoted in the *Chicago Tribune* saying that the Bumbo seat "teaches babies incorrect postural alignment, with a rounded back and the head leaning forward." Our daughter's physical therapist also advised against it.

❑ **Doorway Jumper**

Bouncy swings you suspend from the ceiling, doorway, or a beam in your house. They're cool and super-fun, but you need to find one that's a safe fit for your home. Installing to a beam is recommended over doorway molding. You can also mount on a sturdy tree outdoors!

❏ **Play Mat**

A reasonably portable cushioned area for your baby to play before she can fully crawl all over the place. If you don't have carpet, you'll need this.

An extraordinary number of options are out there. A big, padded rubber mat may be easier to wipe down than a cute puzzle-piece one. Also, it's a pain to clean and reassemble the rubber pieces that have a grooved texture on one side and a porous surface on the other. The pores like to collect all kinds of hairs, dust, and crumbs that prove impossible to get out. Take my word for it.

❏ **Activity Center**

A tent-like structure with a hanging mobile, where you can lay your newborn to play, rest, and wonder, before he is able to move around on his own. It's a great place for you to entertain Baby and also for him to amuse himself while you do your thing.

TAKING BABY FROM A TO Z

❏ **Baby Carrier**

Probably inspired by marsupials, this is a sling or backpack-like contraption you strap your baby into so you can carry her while keeping your arms free to do chores. Yay, women's lib! I kid. Carriers are very popular with dads, too. You can't have enough of them: one in the car, one at the office, one at the house...they're AMAZING. They're the best thing to happen since hands-free car phones.

Take a few brands out for a test ride to find the best one for you. I'm a huge fan of the Ergobaby and the

Baby Björn. I got both of them, along with a Maya wrap, which I never figured out how to safely use (according to the diagram it came with, the sideways position I commonly see it used for is not good for Baby's spine). I loved the Björn because my daughter could face forward and totally engage with the world outside my boobs. We used it exclusively until she surpassed the recommended height and weight, at which point we transitioned to the Ergobaby, a hand-me-down from our neighbor, which does have an infant insert available.

❏ Car Seat

If you have a car, you'll need a car seat. This is the only safe way to transport a child in a vehicle. It is *not* a place where your child should nap/sleep for prolonged periods, as it could lead to positional asphyxia. (Refer to the BIG NO-NO box on page 129 for additional information.)

If you don't end up getting a Snap-N-Go system (more on that below), go for a convertible car seat that grows with your child. We're using the Evenflo Symphony DLX, and so far, so good. We've also used the Maxi Cosi Pria 70 to our satisfaction.

A used car seat is safe as long as you check into

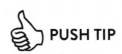 **PUSH TIP**

Installation Is Everything

Proper car seat installation is vital. Contact your local fire department, study the DMV's instructional videos, or hire a professional to install it.

Install the car seat facing the rear and sustain that position for as long as possible. It's the safest.

its lifespan, the manufacturer's recommended height and weight requirements, and make sure it has never been in an accident, as this can make it lose effectiveness. Even too many trips down the baggage claim conveyor belt at the airport can negatively impact a car seat's composition.

❏ **Car Seat Liner**

An easy-to-wash waterproof liner that helps keep your car seat clean. Pretty cheap and totally worth it.

❏ **Car Window Sun Shade**

A shade that suctions to your car window to filter or block sunlight. My retractable screen doesn't do much in the way of "shading," so I make my daughter wear a hat if the sun is blasting. Tinted windows, though costlier, are probably more effective.

❏ **Snap-N-Go Stroller or Stroller Travel System**

A stroller that allows you to snap its associated infant car seat directly into the base. This makes the car/stroller transition super-smooth. You don't even have to wake Baby from a nap when you pull up to where you're going. You just click her off the base of the car seat and onto the legs of your stroller.

I loved our Uppa Baby Cruz and Denny Car Seat Snap-N-Go combo (designed for infants 4 to 35 pounds and up to 32 inches tall). My daughter rode in this for eighteen months. But as our babies get heavier and we get older, the *easy* snap-n-go experience can throw out one's back.

Some travel systems also come equipped with a stroller-compatible bassinet, which may be useful for safe napping. However, I've noticed that for some reason many babies don't like to lie flat when in a stroller.

❑ **Lightweight Stroller**
A compact stroller for when your baby gets older (most are not recommended for infants). Look for a light one that reclines all the way flat for cozy naps, has storage underneath, and that you can easily fold one-handed. I wish I had put this on my registry because when I needed it, I couldn't bring myself to $pend on it. So...I snatched a used one from a fellow mom for five bucks!

❑ **Jogging Stroller**
A stroller with pneumatic tires, perfect for rough terrain or to push while you jog. Definitely invest if you're a runner or expect to "off-road" a lot with your baby.
  You can find many "used" jogging strollers in mint condition from moms who thought they would run but seldom (if ever!) got around it.

❑ **Stroller Seat Liner**
A liner that fits most strollers. Some are designed with special fabrics that keep your baby cool. If you live in a hot area or your baby is prone to "explosions," this may be worth acquiring.

❑ **Stroller Sleep Sack**
A cozy sleeping bag that straps into most strollers to keep Baby warm. Put on your registry if you live anywhere other than Puerto Rico or California—you know: places that experience seasons.

❑ **Stroller Wrist Strap**
A safety harness to prevent the stroller from rolling away from you. This is particularly handy if you live in a hilly area. Always insist that caregivers use it, too—I can't

tell you how many nannies I see strolling downhill with one hand on the stroller and the other typing into their phones. It brings out the tiger mom in me. *Roar.*

❑ **Shopping Cart and High Chair Covers**
If you're a bit of a germaphobe, this may be your ticket to taking kiddo to the grocery store or the local bistro pub. I didn't get one because I'm okay with a few germs and didn't want to add to my laundry pile.

❑ **Disposable Changing Pads**
A basic for any diaper bag, disposable liners are sort of like toilet-seat covers, to be used in public changing stations. Breastfed newborn poop likes to spill over, so using these at home, too, saved us time and water. We loved Daddy's disposable changing pads from Daddy & Co.

Disposable stuff adds up in our landfills, so I tried to be considerate. My thrifty ass reused liners 'til they were soiled, and even then, I would cut out the pooped-on part to reuse the rest.

❑ **Diaper Bag**
A bag with lots of compartments to transport your baby's paraphernalia. Unless you have many hands like Ganesha, this is kind of a must. We got the backpack kind and I liked it, but my husband didn't. In retrospect, I should've asked him to weigh in. Because he was embarrassed to tote a bright blue-and-green diaper bag, he avoided it at all costs—at my expense! My hip friends settled for a vintage camera bag, which is both multipurpose and gender neutral.

Diaper Bag Survival Kit

- Diapers (3–5 per child)
- Wipes (with built-in lid)
- Sunblock
- Sun hat
- Beanie (if in cold weather)
- Extra clothes for Baby (don't forget socks!) *and* for you
- Bug repellent
- Bib
- Portable placemat if Baby is old enough to eat solids
- Plastic bags (Ziplocs or biodegradable poop bags)
- Any kind of blanket you can purpose as a nursing cover, sunshade, changing pad, or burp cloth
- Small first-aid kit, including Infants' Tylenol
- Toiletry bag: moisturizer, diaper rash cream, nipple cream
- Quick-change bag: a mini bag stocked with a diaper and wipes for changes on the go without having to tote the whole shebang
- Bottled water (to drink and/or mix with formula powder)
- Formula powder or pre-mixed formula bottle (even if you are exclusively breastfeeding, it could be handy in an emergency)
- Snacks (for you, and Baby if old enough)
- Duplicate of Baby's favorite book and/or toy
- Spare pacifier
- Reading material (for you)
- Extra cash, change, or credit card

CHILDPROOFING & MONITORING

❏ **Childproofing Products**

Babyproofing doomsday is looming and there are many things to secure in a home: electronics, household cleaners, knives, furniture, outlets...pretty much anything that can cut, choke, suffocate, poison, electrocute, or squish your child will need to be secured.

Here's a list of items you could potentially need down the line:

❏ Finger pinch door guards (to keep from slamming doors on little fingers)

❏ Doorknob covers

❏ Stove knob guards

❏ Window guards

❏ Sliding door stickers (so your child doesn't walk into it)

❏ Electrical outlet plugs (buy the largest ones available, as these can be a choking hazard)

❏ Cord stops and safety tassels (to keep appliance cords and curtain cords away from your child for fear of electrocution, strangling, or getting hit with what's on the other end of the cord)

❏ Fireplace grill

❏ Drawer and cabinet locks or latches (adhesive magnetic ones are very popular these days)

❏ Refrigerator lock or latch

❏ Appliance- and furniture-anchoring straps and latches

❏ Pool fence

❑ Coffee table corner guards

❑ Toilet-lid locks

❑ Soft cover for bath faucet (so baby doesn't bump his head on it)

❑ Non-slip bath mat

❑ Safety gates and banister guards (for stairs)

Childproofing can be a gradual process or an intensive weekend project. We went for gradual and the hovering helicopter approach. As previously disclosed, our home is only minimally rigged with babyproofing gadgets. Call me a whirlybird all you want, but no gadget is a substitute for supervising my child.

As far as the registry, not many people find cabinet locks cute enough to gift and you won't need this stuff for a while, so you may be on your own.

❑ **Baby Monitor**

A device that allows you to listen and maybe even see your child while they're in a different room—and if you get a *really* fancy one, from a faraway land. If you live in a studio apartment or are planning on co-sleeping, you may not need a monitor. Also, these devices are essentially radio transmitters, meaning other monitors nearby can pick up your signal, which creeps me out a bit. But it didn't stop me from getting one.

We recently forgot our monitor when took our daughter on a trip to my in-laws, and I felt like the worst mother on the planet. But you know what? We could hear her crying just fine without it. That said, we love ours and would admittedly be stressed without it.

Here's what to look for in a monitor:

✓ **Video.** A very nice feature, though not entirely necessary. I did like to be able to see my daughter's belly go up and down during those (paranoid) early days.

✓ **Pan/tilt functionality.** Your baby will move around the crib and if you've got the video feature, you'll want to be able to find her.

✓ **Wall mount.** So you can mount the camera out of reach. If your child is like ours, she'll be trying to find and destroy big brother in the middle of the night.

✓ **Separate power cords.** One for the monitor and one for the camera. Otherwise you can't charge both at the same time.

✓ **Speaker/walkie-talkie capability.** So you can tell Junior that you're on your way, or that he needs to go back to sleep for a little longer.

✓ **Sensor pad.** A pad you place underneath the mattress to monitor Baby's breathing and movement. This could ease your mind, but they are pricey and I've read mixed reviews. Some parents complain that the sensors are too sensitive, so the "alarm" wakes up the baby—and parents.

✓ **Live streaming.** If you travel a lot or work long hours, consider investing in a video monitor or system such as NEST that streams to your phone, so you can always spy on the nanny. Err, monitor your baby.

✓ **Zoom.** Worth it only if your camera is mounted far away from your baby.

✓ **Musical feature.** We haven't used it, but many parents like it. I find it annoying because you hear the darn music through the receiver, too.

✓ **Charge capacity.** Don't get anything that lasts under six hours—you want something that stays charged longer than your baby sleeps! (Another reason why two different power cords are key.)

✓ **Easy-to-replace parts.** I can't find a replacement power adapter for my model *anywhere*. Since my daughter dropped it, I've spent about twenty minutes each night finding the right angle to make it stay plugged in. It's maddening.

❑ **Car Seat Mirror**

A mirror that attaches to the headrest across from your baby's rear-facing car seat. The reflection (your baby) can be seen in the rearview mirror, as well as vice-versa, so you and your baby can check on each other while you drive. Of course, it can be distracting. Who wants to look at the road when there's a cute baby in the back?! I'm guilty as charged.

BATH TIME

❑ **Baby Bathtub**

My mom used to bathe me in the kitchen sink. We've come a long way since then, and you can now purchase several types of products to help you cleanse your baby. We ended up buying two.

We started out with the Angelcare Baby Bath Support. This is great if you will be using it in a shower. I'm still a fan, but you waste a lot of water if you use it soak-style inside a tub. Also, once our baby started sitting up, she could no longer safely use this device; a few times I saved her from face-planting onto the tub, which was another strike against it.

We then had to cough up the cash for a Stokke Flexi Bath and we absolutely loved it. It folds neatly so you can store it after use. And you can get a Flexi Bath Newborn Support insert for those first months.

I've since become aware of the Tummy Tub and the Wash Pod, which are bucket tubs that help babies assume fetal position (sitting upright) while in the bath. You can purchase stands for them to avoid kneeling while bathing your baby.

Some important things to look for in a tub: contains infant insert or is infant-appropriate; non-skid; easy to rinse and dry; drain stop; and ease of storage (foldable). In terms of built-in water temperature readers, I'm skeptical of sticker gauges, but I have read that digital readers are pretty accurate. We were fine without this feature and if you can trust your good ol' hand to make sure the water's not too hot, you may not need it either.

❑ **Knee Pad or Gardening Pad**
A cushion to kneel on while you bathe your baby—you'll need this! My friend gifted me one and her card read: "So you'll think of me every time you're on your knees." Best. Line. Ever.

❑ **Hooded Bath Towel**
Towel with a built-in hoodie so your baby's nugget stays warm and dry after bath. Pick something super soft and cuddly.

❏ **Washcloth or Sponge**
You'll need one of these to scrub your baby clean. My baby is totally sponge-worthy. (Please refer to *Seinfeld* Season 7 "The Sponge.") However, if you go for the sponge, keep in mind that it can break apart and pose a choking hazard. Washcloths are safer and have a longer life span.

❏ **Baby Shampoo or Body Wash**
Because the skin is our biggest organ, it's worth investing in high-quality products. Your registry is a good way to test an expensive brand on someone else's dime!

FOR SOOTHING, WELL-BEING, & GROOMING

❏ **Blankets & Swaddlers**
Blankets come in a variety of colors, textures, and sizes, each claiming to have a different purpose. I found them to be fairly interchangeable, but here are some specific types:

❏ **Receiving Blankets** are general-use lightweight blankets, historically used for parents to "receive" a baby after birth. They're designed to keep Baby warm, but can be used for many purposes, including a burp cloth, a sleep shade, an on-the-go changing mat, a boob-sweat wipe— you name it.
    You'll probably get a ton of these whether you register for them or not, but it's nice to select some favorites that go with your décor.

❏ **Burp Cloths** are used to wipe up spit. You can use just about anything to wipe up spit, and in fact, you *will* use just about anything, because you'll never have your official burp cloth at hand when you need it.

❑ **Swaddling Blankets, Wearable Blankets, Sleep Sacks, & Sleepsuits** are created specially to help your baby feel snug and soothe him to sleep. We loved the aden + anais blankets, but the "silky soft swaddles" were too soft for baby-wrapping, causing the "burrito" to come undone. The classic ones are stiffer and better for a snug cocoon.

Be forewarned that swaddling is a magician's art and your baby is a little Houdini. Once he learns to finagle his way out of your origami burrito, you may need a specialized sleepsuit or wearable blanket. When our daughter refused to stay in a swaddle at five months, we became loyalists of the Merlin Sleepsuit, which we used until she was one. It was a bit stuffy—she looked like the Stay Puft Marshmallow Man from *Ghostbusters* in it—so on hot nights, we used an aden + anais wearable blanket.

❑ **Pacifier**
These can be well worth having if they effectively soothe your crying baby. However, not all kids take to them and if they do, it's sometimes hard to wean them off them down the line.

Always be sure the nipple is not chewed off—you don't want it breaking and your baby choking, or even swallowing a piece.

❑ **Teething Toys**
You'll find a variety of teething toys, rings, and sticks made out of wood, rubber, and plastic to help your baby scratch their gums. We loved the Baby Banana Bendable Training Toothbrush. Our daughter went nuts over it and we think it helped her get used to a real toothbrush. We

also loved their Bendable Animal Teethers made with medical-grade non-toxic silicone. Our daughter never took to the gel/cold ones, but those can be good, too. Parents love the cute Sophie Giraffe, a French-made toy composed of rubber and food-grade paint, but we never gave it a try because we're cheapskates. And if, like me, you want to feel better about not spending the money, search for images of "moldy Sophie Giraffe." *Oh là là.*

Teething toys are always a nice "add-on" to a registry, as people like to "round up" their gift. My moms club recently had an email thread on teethers and the two that stood out were ARK's Z-Vibes (it's pricey but our daughter's occupational therapist recommended it to try to help her latch) and Bobbins Lullaby maple wood washable teether from Etsy. You can also find teethers made out of cornstarch resin or silicone.

❏ **Snot Extractor**
Different devices to help clear your baby's nasal passage of snot. These help your baby breathe when he is congested. But beware that over-"sucking" can dry out and cause inflammation in the nasal passages.

❏ The **Bulb Syringe** has been around for ages. It's a suctioning device you insert into the nostril to extract boogies. We chose this option, making sure to replace it periodically, as those things can be a Petri dish for mold.

❏ The **NoseFrida** is reportedly more effective, but there's no way in hell my husband or I was going to suck snot through a straw—even with a catch-all filter. A lot of my less finicky friends love the Frida. Slurp away!

❑ **Humidifier**

A humidifier helps keep the room's atmosphere moist, which helps to relieve baby's congestion if he is sick, and to keep his skin moisturized. If you live in a dry-weather region or have central AC, it's worth adding to your registry. Cold humidifiers are safer, in the event that the water spills. Also, be warned that humidifiers require lots of cleaning and drying to avoid mold growth.

We got the Humio Ultrasonic and we're happy with it, though to Baby the lights are like flames to a moth. This unit has an essential oil compartment as well.

❑ **First-Aid Kit**

Every home and car should have a regular first-aid kit. Additionally, you'll want to add infant's Tylenol, Benadryl, and/or your pain reliever/allergy reducer of choice.

❑ **Thermometer**

Thermometers measure your baby's temperature. An array of products are designed to take a temperature reading in different places: orally, rectally, and axillary.

BIG NØ-NØ!

Avoid Glass and Mercury Thermometers

The old-school glass thermometer is no longer considered safe—even if it has a non-mercury solution inside—as the glass can be easily broken.

145

I've found that all these various devices are hard to operate, inconsistent, and frustrating. I get a different reading each time I take my daughter's temperature with the same the thermometer pressed against her forehead. If you can afford to, buy all three and see which one gives you the most consistent results.

For further details, I've outlined a glossary of thermometers in *Chapter 12: Sick Is a Four-Letter Word.*

❏ **Baby's First Manicure: Nail Scissors, Clippers, & File**
You'll need to keep baby's fingernails trimmed so she doesn't scratch herself or others. We prefer the clippers, but my good friend Mari swears by the scissors. Whatever makes you less nervous about clipping those teeny nails on those precious fingers!! As far as the nail file, I'd love to know if anyone has ever successfully filed their newborn's nails.

❏ **Baby Brush**
If your baby has hair, you'll want to brush it. (Also, congrats! Mine looked like Friar Tuck for almost a year.) You'll find a variety of soft-bristled brushes to choose from.

BABY WEAR

❏ **PJs**
PJs are my favorite cozy thing to buy for babies. I find zippers easier to deal with than snaps, but this is a matter of preference. When registering for PJs, list a variety of sizes, and keep in mind that for six months and up you may need no-slip footies. Kids need the traction once they start to crawl, stand, and walk.

I'm a big fan of using previously loved PJs and also of donating them to nonprofit organizations that service women, children, and the homeless.

❏ **Onesies**

Your baby will live in a onesie for the first few months of life. You're bound to get a surplus of them, so if you're particular and want to make sure they span a few sizes, put them on your registry. Keep in mind that newborn (NB) sizes don't fit a lot of babies. My daughter was 8 pounds, 6 ounces and never fit into any of the NB stuff she got.

❏ **T-Shirts**

You'll get so many clothes, I advocate keeping them off the registry. Unlike onesies, your baby will wear T-shirts more often when he's older and you've come to loathe the extra step of snapping and unsnapping buttons during a change.

❏ **Leggings or Pull-Ons**

Same as T-shirts, though you may use them over onesies if it's cold outside. We live in California and she was born in summer, so she lived pantless for months.

❏ **Socks & Booties**

The more, the merrier. You go through these fast! The best booties EVER are Zutano's. They stay on!

❏ **Hats**

Register for weather-appropriate hats for sunny days, rainy days, and snowy days in different sizes.

❏ **Scratch-Free Mittens**

Lightweight mittens that prevent babies from scratching themselves while they sleep. I tried a few pairs on my daughter, but they never stayed on. Luckily, she wasn't a big scratcher, but some kids are. I recommend buying or registering for at least one pair because they *can* come in (ready for it?) *handy!*

❏ **Snowsuit & Mittens**

If you live where it's cold, this is a very good idea. Get something that will last a while size-wise, keeping in mind the date of your baby's birth and the upcoming seasons (i.e., if your baby is born in the summer, it won't get cold 'til he's about six months old).

Snowsuits in particular can be pricey and are quickly outgrown. If you miss the registry boat, I would try to find something used in your mom community.

ENTERTAINMENT

❏ **Toys**

If there's a specific or expensive toy you can't live without, by all means add it to your registry. But toy chests grow with your kid and it's best to keep them "pruned."

I purge every so often and donate previously loved items to charity. I'm always on the lookout for hand-me-downs as well!

❏ **Books**

We're big fans. You may want to buy or put on your registry a few collector's item first editions of childhood classics such as *Alice in Wonderland*; just be sure to safeguard them until your baby is old enough not to destroy them.

We're also into used books and borrowing from our local library.

GOODIES FOR MOM

❑ **Post-Pregnancy Shapewear**

Designed to help you tame your tummy back to its former self. I used Belly Bandit and had a great experience. They make a variety of "wear" beyond the belly band: control tops, leggings, corsets...you name it. Find the brand for you and shrink away.

❑ **Spirits**

I mean the drinking kind. Wine and beer included. Put a wine club on your registry—maybe someone will gift Mama her therapy cocktail.

❑ **Food Delivery Service**

Many companies are set up to bring you prepped or catered meals. Register for a gift certificate to one of your choosing. Your loved ones can also help you set up a food delivery schedule in your community or through a company like Meal Train. I was too proud to ask, but I'd have killed for a home-cooked meal (not by me) those first few weeks. One night a few days after pushing, I cooked salmon, roasted potatoes, and brussels sprouts for my family. But mainly, we survived on pizza and pad thai.

❑ **Babysitting Coupons**

IOUs people can give you for a night off. *Hells, yeah!* You can even outline special dates on the registry when you would love to cash in on some babysitting. The con: You may get Auntie Smokie volunteering for a shift.

The gang of misfits attending your shower notwithstanding, what's more soothing than free help? *Well, maybe...(see next)...*

❏ **Massage Gift Certificates**

I wish I had registered for these. Your entire body will go to shit during pregnancy. Your back, your hips, your wrists, your neck. You'll absolutely need a massage, but if you're cheap like me, you'll find it hard to justify the expense. See if someone else will help you get there guilt-free! Best. Gift. Ever.

GIFTS THAT KEEP ON GIVING

❏ **Parent Group Membership and/or Parent and Me Classes**
Receiving an activity gift to bond with your baby is so green!

For months, I thought I was too cool to join a mom group or anything that involved a team of sleepless mothers singing "Kumbaya" with their kids in a circle. But I promise that you'll find a kindred spirit who will laugh appreciatively when you mutter: "Shit, I forgot to feed the meter" in the middle of *"The wheels on the bus go round and round, round and round..."* Mom groups can be lifesavers when you need advice, product recommendations, solace, validation, hand-me-downs, or just a safe place to share your woes. Going in to motherhood, I didn't perceive moms as "cool" people. I'm happy to report I was very wrong. I've met some of the coolest ladies in my mom community.

Most support groups will be specific to your area. In East L.A., I found nonprofit mom clubs with a small annual fee, and a wide array of Parent and Me classes, some activity-based, some geared towards different developmental stages.

Parent-support hubs such as The Pump Station offer great classes and also a convenient place to feed and change your baby. I really loved visiting The Pump Station while out running errands during those early months.

❏ **Gift Cards**
To any store. And since not everyone can afford big gifts, putting multiple gift cards of small denominations on your registry gives friends the opportunity to chip in for a big-ticket item.

❏ **Subscription Services**
Paid subscription programs such as Amazon Prime reissue your monthly staples (diapers, vitamins, household supplies) at a discount and free of shipping costs. Prime also comes with a video streaming service, so you get free entertainment to boot!

Baby Shower Confidential

Having a shower goes hand in hand with creating a registry. It's the occasion in which you get to showcase your bounty in front of your favorite friends and relatives (as well as obligatory invitees!). Being showered in celebration of the baby growing inside of you is one of the most amazing perks of being pregnant. Here are a few tips to help you be a rock star at your own baby shower.

#1 *Be considerate*

Don't turn into a shower-zilla and demand that only Dom Pérignon be served with cold-pressed organic grapefruit juice. Be considerate of everyone's financial situation and don't put things on your registry that only a Kardashian could afford; poor Aunt Jo will feel awful that she can only buy you a burp cloth, and if you open your gifts in front of the crowd, everyone will witness the disparity.

Although a baby shower is meant to help lessen the financial burden of a new mom, the most important takeaway is to establish a support system for this stage in your life.

#2 *Don't be a backseat driver*

Of course you want to give direction for your shower. You may want to give input regarding the color scheme, centerpieces, themes, location, time of day—it is absolutely your right. You can even start a Pinterest board with your host. But do know when to step back and let the host have some fun, too. This is different in every case: some hosts will want to be more involved than others. It's up to you to feel it out and be involved as much or as little as needed.

#3 *Be classy*

I've thrown a few showers, and they can get pricey. If you can (and especially if the host is not affluent), it may be nice to offer to shoulder some of the cost, bring some of the food, take on the favors, pay for the location, provide the booze, buy the flowers, or make some of the decorations. If you do offer, make sure you stay true to your word and pay up. I've been in situations where I went overbudget, thinking someone would chip in, and they didn't. It wasn't a big deal, but I do know of another instance where it got awkward. Nobody wants to be fighting over receipts.

If possible, try to arrive a little early to help set up and decorate—even if the host insists they don't need you. Every shower I've ever hosted has been a race to the very last minute.

#4 *Be grateful*

Gift your hosts with a token of your gratitude. Also, mail personal and thoughtful thank-you notes to guests soon after the shower. Which brings me to the next little tip...

#5 *Make it easier on you*

You'll need plenty of thank-you cards to thank everyone. If a close friend or relative is throwing your shower, maybe secretly ask if she could set up a table with labels so people can write their own address for you to simply peel, stick, and mail. Stamping the envelopes with postage is a plus. Of course, the host should take all the credit! ☺

(P.S. Have her read this book. She'll take the hint.)

Now that we've covered all the bases of baby showers and registering, let's go back to the question at hand: *Do* you really need all this crap for a teeny-weeny baby? Honestly, no. All you need at first are diapers, wipes, a few blankets, bottles, a safe place for baby to sleep, a car seat if you have a car, a fairly big supply of onesies, and a huge surplus of unconditional, patient, endless love. That's it. No need to break the bank. You can make your kitchen sink a tub, the best teething toys are often wooden spoons, and no mobile is better than your own two hands backed by your very own lullabies.

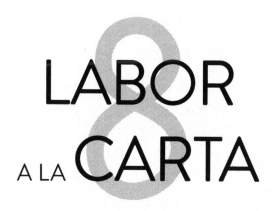

LABOR
A LA CARTA

Eeny, Meeny, Miny, Moe...
Mi Mamá Picks the Very Best One

MANY A PREGNANT NIGHT, I lay in bed with a memory foam pillow jammed between my unshaven legs, staring at the red glare of the clock's numbers bouncing off the wall, ruminating over every single choice I had to make in order to bring this baby into the world. I knew I would try to deliver in a hospital, but I had to decide: *Do I take birth classes? Do I hire a doula? Do I bank the baby's cord? Do I encapsulate my placenta?* The anxiety seed within me was sprouting like a weed—and I didn't even have to factor in circumcision!

Nobody had told me that preparing for delivery would be harder than studying for the multiple-choice logic section of the SAT. I almost wished I was one of those women on TV who didn't know they were pregnant until they went into labor. Then I could've avoided the ticking of that decision-making clock that comes with a baby growing in your belly.

I'm talking about all the technical options and alternative courses of action that require research and soul-searching, and inevitably come with unsolicited judgment from family and friends. Thankfully, my husband was cool with anything I wanted—as long as it didn't involve him standing in the line of fire. This was amazingly supportive of him. (And I say this without an ounce of sarcasm—I didn't want him to have a front-row seat, either.) However, his being so agreeable left *me* to call all the shots.

I researched every option, obsessed over every possibility, and drove my husband crazy along the way. He, in turn, drove me insane with his "Whatever you want, baby." I hope to spare you and your partner's time and sanity with the intel I collected.

In a perfect world, each labor would come with its own menú a la carta. So I've tried my best to lay it all out. *Buen provecho!*

Birth 101: Attend or Cut Class?

Birth classes are either for you or not.

Are you a recipe-follower or do you like to improvise in the kitchen?

When I cook, I like to skim a few recipes, chuck them, come up with my own, and then burn myself trying to replicate what I just absorbed. In all seriousness, I'm a classified "intuitive learner." I do best when I'm thrown into situations where I have to find my way as I go along. And when I do, I'm usually unable to tell you how I got there. Needless to say, I'm a poor student in the traditional sense.

If you're more of a sensing learner, one who thrives on familiarity and succeeds with facts, training, and practice—or simply a curious being who gets a kick out of new experiences—then a birth class is a must.

And, yes, you absolutely *can* still take a class to prepare you for a C-section. In fact, a lot of birth classes that favor vaginal delivery also simulate an emergency C-section to help you prepare for how you'll feel on the other side of the silk screen.

Some classes also make the non-birthing partner take the "hot seat," so they can be more empathetic throughout the process. These sort of rehearsal drills make both my husband and me very anxious, so we decided to skip birth class altogether.

Assuming you're a bit less self-conscious than we are, a labor and birth course could help both you and your partner feel prepared and confident going into delivery.

WHERE TO ENROLL

A myriad of birth classes are offered by various community hubs: moms clubs, yoga studios, clinics, and more. To ensure an objective perspective, you may want to explore independent options that are not in any way affiliated with a specific hospital, birth center, or doula service. Be wary of anyone trying to sell you on something that doesn't feel right to you.

That said, if you're absolutely certain of the kind of birthing experience you're seeking to accomplish, do book a class with your preferred labor alliance.

To Push or Not to Push?

For us first world humans, being born is probably the most dangerous day of our lives. Any kind of birth involves risks. A vaginal birth can be a powerful experience for many a woman, but it's not for every woman. And in a free society, a woman has the right to be supported in her choice of delivery method, whatever it may be.

My mom had three Cesarean sections in less than four years—and this was back when a woman's stomach was split from the belly button down to the pubic bone. But the scar my mother bore scarred *me* for life. Thankfully, science has come a long way and the Cesarean cicatrix is no longer a big issue. Many women even schedule a bikini wax and mani/pedi before their C-section. There's nothing wrong with getting your pubes yanked before going under the knife.

For many, this decision is a no-brainer. For others, it can be a bit of a mind-grater. When considering your options, do a risk/benefit analysis with your doctor to help determine what will work best for you.

VAGINAL DELIVERY: PROS & CONS

If you're willing and able to push your baby, a vaginal delivery has huge benefits.

Perhaps the biggest one is to your baby. As a baby comes through the birth canal, his lungs are squeezed of fluids that could cause breathing complications down the line. Also, the birthing journey from the womb into the cervix and through the vagina exposes your child to good bacteria that boosts a newborn's immune system and protects his intestinal tract—even if that journey sounds comparable to crawling through a sewer line.

Sometimes, to reduce risks during a vaginal delivery, doctors recommend labor induction. (Not to give anything away, but you can read all about it in the next chapter, *Chapter 9: We Make Plans and God Laughs at Our Vaginas: My Birthing Story: A Page-One Rewrite.*) This "induced" advice may go against your plans, so to help you navigate these waters, I consulted a Fellow on the American Board of Oriental Reproductive Medicine, who is a Licensed Acupuncturist and Herbalist with a Master's Degree in Traditional Chinese Medicine.

Here is some helpful information she shared:

SOME QUESTIONS TO CONSIDER WHEN YOUR DOCTOR SAYS: "LET'S GET THIS BABY OUTTA HERE"

by Abigail Morgan, L.Ac, FABORM, Founder/Owner of FLOAT: Chinese Medical Arts in Glendale, CA, Mother of Two

Medical induction can be a lifesaver for Mom and Baby under some circumstances. However, it is not always the safest option for either. Post-date pregnancy is NOT a reason for medical induction until the forty-first week of pregnancy.

Here are some important questions to discuss with your OB/GYN when and if medical induction is recommended:

1. For what reasons are you recommending induction?

2. What are the risks associated with inducing now vs. waiting until I go into labor on my own?

3. Is my baby having heart decelerations?

4. What is my Bishop score? (Also known as a cervix score, this is a system that assesses your odds of spontaneous delivery.)

5. Do you have any concerns about my using non-medical approaches to try to get labor to start naturally? (E.g., acupuncture, intercourse, castor oil, walking...)

6. How will you induce me? (E.g., using a prostaglandin gel such as Cervidil or Cytotec [misoprostol], a balloon catheter, Pitocin, breaking my water, etc.)

7. What are the possible side effects of your intended measures and medications?

Any procedure must be offered to you under what is called Informed Consent. Administering a procedure (induction or anything else) without permission is considered battery of a patient and can be grounds for the loss of the doctor's license.

The relationship between an OB/GYN and her patient (the pregnant mama) should be a partnership; a patient must feel heard, respected, and trusted to make her own informed decisions.

Your doctor may be the expert in the care of a fetus and the management of a pregnancy, but you are in charge of your body. You get to be included in all decision-making about what happens to it. This is true choice.

Induced or not, an uncomplicated vaginal delivery presents few risks for baby, though some are plausible. For example, bruised scalps or fractured collarbones are more common in children born vaginally, occurring when the baby is big or after a prolonged labor.

When it comes to literally pushing your baby into this world, some experts suggest for women to only push when the urge arises— a strategy used commonly in communities that favor unassisted birth. And it does make sense: Most babies will travel down with ease once they're ready to come out. A push-when-you-want-to program was implemented at Medway Maritime Hospital in the UK, and the incidence of severe vaginal tearing decreased significantly. Overpushing can also result in tailbone or pelvic injury. So if you find yourself amongst a circle of people yelling "Push!", feel free to tell them: "This is my party and I'll push if I want to."

After a vaginal birth, if all goes smoothly, Mom can hold and breastfeed Baby (if preferred). And usually her body recovers faster. I say "usually" because I know a set of sisters who gave birth at about the same time. One pushed and the other had a C-section. The sister with the C-section was up and running way before her younger sister, who (as the C-sister put it) "tore the shit out of her vagina."

I don't mean to scare you, but having a baby will probably hurt no matter what kind of delivery you have. And many gloss over the effects of a vaginal delivery. Pushing, alone, can cause broken pelvis bones or injury, a prolapsed uterus (when the pelvic floor muscles stretch too far and the uterus droops into the vagina), and severe tears, which can lead to bacterial infection, incontinence, nerve pain, and/or numbness.

Your fanny (British for vagina) is an important factor to consider in choosing your own labor adventure. She will be exposed to a lot more "uncontrolled" damage with vaginal delivery, which could possibly take a lot longer to heal than a C-section incision. Conversely, a C-section may disrupt harmony in your internal organs. No matter what, you could get beat.

Tears Over Tears

When giving birth, you may suffer varying tears or lacerations around the labia and/or inside the vagina. Be assured that tears (and your tears over them!) aren't permanent—you will eventually recover.

Labia tears are known to be fairly painful and they range from superficial scrapes to, well, actual tears.

If you get what's known as a **vaginal or perineal tear** on your perineum (the area between the vulva and anus), you'll get to enjoy one of four different levels of badness:

Level 1: Superficial tearing of the skin or the vaginal area.

Level 2: Tearing of the muscles surrounding the vagina.

Level 3: Vaginal tear that extends through perineum and outer sphincter muscles, stopping at the inner lining of your anus, called the rectal mucosa. (In other words, it breaches the "outer ring" of your anus, but not the "inner ring"—yes, your-anus has rings!)

Level 4: This tear progresses beyond the anal sphincter and may cause a total rupture of the rectal mucosa. (This creates what's known to some as a "vaganus"—because your anus is basically now conjoined with your vagina.)

C-SECTION: PROS & CONS

For a myriad of medical reasons, a C-section is the safest option for many women and their babies. If you suffer from placenta previa (your placenta is blocking the birth canal), your baby is breech or tied up in the umbilical cord, or either you or your baby has a medical condition that could be exacerbated by a vaginal delivery, a Cesarean section may be your only option. Some doctors also recommend this procedure based on the mother's age and medical history. And if you're having twins or your baby is very large, a C-section may be recommended as it could carry the least amount of risk.

In a recent discussion amongst moms who had undergone medically advised C-sections, many bonded over the understanding that hundreds of years ago, they might have died in childbirth. In fact, as my friend's 4'1" grandmother was pushing an eleven-pound baby out of her hoo-ha, she was told matter-of-factly that she wasn't going to make it. I'm happy to report that *Abuelita* did survive, but the point is, it was *that* commonplace for women to die during labor.

Please note, though: Sound evidence exists that some doctors prefer this procedure over pushing because it's time-efficient and the outcome is more predictable—which can also be desirable to many women. But you don't want the C-decision to be made for you for the wrong reasons. Seek a second opinion if you don't feel comfortable with your doctor's recommendation.

For those considering an optional C-section, a scheduled birth is appealing to any devout planner out there: you pick the date and time, and you are ensured that your vagina will survive intact. Though your abdominal area may not.

During a C-section, your abdomen and uterus are sliced open to extract your baby from the womb. Your uterus, along with its fallopian tubes, may be temporarily removed outside your body. Some other organs may also be pushed around inside of you. In rare instances, your intestines may be harmed and pulled out for repair, or your uterus could rupture. Your baby may also get nicked along the way. A C-section also increases chances of Mom contracting an infection, getting a blood clot, or suffering an organ injury.

The maternal mortality rate is higher with a Cesarean than a vaginal birth. So the bottom line is: a C-section is generally riskier than a vaginal delivery for both Mom and Baby.

Also, with a C-section, you may have to wait twenty to thirty minutes to hold your baby, and it may take up to an hour until you're able nurse. However, this has not shown to be detrimental to the ability to breastfeed in the long run or affect a mom's connection to her baby.

Finally, some women who get C-sections complain that they didn't feel as though they were a part of their own delivery experience. Very recently, to address this, some practitioners provide a small tent-like opening in the sheet set up to block the field of vision between a woman and her baby-maker. This allows a new mom to peek through the partition and see her child coming out of her womb, which may help her feel more connected to the experience. If this sounds like just the thing for you, don't be afraid to ask for it.

The Birth of the Successful C-Section

C-section operations have been performed since antiquity to dead or dying mothers in hopes of saving their child.

The first recorded Cesarean in which mother and child both survived was in Switzerland in the 1500s when swine-gelder Jacob Nufer sliced his wife open, removed the baby, and stitched her back up.

In the U.S., an effective C-section didn't happen until 1794, when Jesse Bennett took over his wife's difficult childbirth after the attending doctor refused to perform surgery on her. Under duress, Jesse gave laudanum to his wife, Elizabeth, and made the cut. He saved Mom and Baby Maria, but not without purposely removing his wife's ovaries. Let's just say the birth control pill wasn't available at the time!

For you trivia mavens: Maria grew up to bear six children of her own.

WHEN PLAN B IS PLAN C(-SECTION)

Sometimes, the road to a C-section is paved with birth intentions. When "push comes to shove," sudden complications may pressure you to go under the knife, even if you don't want to. Amidst the throes of labor, your doctor may recommend a C-section in order to prevent certain unfavorable outcomes and, yes, liabilities. This is usually referred to as an "emergency C-section."

As much as it's your right to get a second opinion, if you trust your doctor, heed her advice, especially during a time-critical situation. If a true emergency happens—and it *can* happen—remember that becoming a mother *is* the experience. Pushing a baby out of your vagina isn't motherhood. It doesn't make you a better mom, a finer woman, or qualify you as a superhero. Bringing a healthy baby into this world is the end game; so don't risk your baby's well-being or your own because you really want to push.

As Dr. Amy Tuteur, author of *The Skeptical OB,* puts it: "A birth that results in a live, healthy baby and live, healthy mother is inherently superior, and for a significant proportion of women, that birth is a Cesarean section" (*Time* magazine, October 12, 2011).

No doubt there are many great benefits to vaginal delivery—I chose it and was lucky to be able to follow through with my plan without too much collateral damage; but a proud C-mama with a happy, healthy C-baby and unscathed vagina is equally amazing in my book.

ENJOYING THE C-RIDE (THE SECOND TIME AROUND)

by Adrienne M., TV Editor, Los Angeles, CA, Mother of Two

I was definitely having a vaginal birth. I had prepared my whole life for the chance to let my body do what it was meant to do: open up and bring forth a child in the beautiful miracle of a birth, free of drugs or medical intervention. Women have been doing it for all of history and survived. Well, except for all those who died in the process—but I digress...

I was registered at the birthing center and had bantered with the midwives who would guide me through my birth. I was all set.

Until: A couple of weeks before my daughter was due, I rubbed the area just below the bottom of my breastbone and muttered aloud: "Wow, this baby has a big butt!"

Well, it wasn't a big BUTT...

It was a big HEAD. Nice and cozy, tucked right up under my ribs.

A breech baby—me?!

I was devastated. This was not a part of my plan.

I immediately quit my job and set myself to the pressing task of flipping this child. I went to a Chinese acupuncturist and a chiropractor. I burned Moxa sticks by my pinkie toes. I laid upside-down on an ironing board precariously balanced on the couch. My husband once found me at the top of the stairs of our third-floor walk-up, on all fours, head dangling, rolling through some yoga cat-cows. At nine months pregnant, it was more cow than cat.

When none of that worked, we did the mother of all flipping maneuvers: the external cephalic version (ECV). This is when a doctor manually attempts to turn a baby 180 degrees from the outside of your body. Google told me this procedure would be "uncomfortable." It was a few million notches above that. *Is this a glimpse into what childbirth feels like? (Drugs, please!)* My writhes of pain were too much for my husband. I saw his eyes roll backwards over the top of his surgical mask.

"Are you okay?" I asked.

As he replied *"Ummmmm,"* his head dropped onto my chest. He was out cold.

A nurse got him smelling salts and suggested he get prepared for surgery, because my baby hadn't turned. It was time to schedule my C-section.

I immediately started sobbing. I felt like a failure. I mourned the loss of the natural childbirth I had envisioned. I tearfully kissed good-bye the image of rushing to the birth center, managing the labor, the glorious moment of seeing my baby emerge from my body, and then immediately holding her to my chest to nurse in a warm, dimly lit room with my perfectly curated playlist purring in the background.

The sentenced C-section went smoothly, though the pain afterwards was worse than expected (Duh!). My husband was not permitted to sleep over in the room with me, and I spent four long nights navigating my pain alone, struggling with breastfeeding, and feeling sorry for myself.

Three and a half years later, I had my second breech baby girl, born via C-section, too. I went through the same rigmarole trying to turn her, again to no avail. But one thing was very different: I was truly, humbly grateful to deliver my child in a safe, clean, and comparatively low-pain environment. If I had birthed my children in the woods, holding on to a tree like the women in history I had romanticized and admired...I probably would have died—as would have they if their baby was breech—and that would be that. So my body wasn't meant to push big baby heads out. I can *live* with that.

The second time around, I marveled at the beauty of my daughter's shriveled little gray ass being pulled out through the surgical incision in my abdomen. I *did* give birth. I was no less of a woman or mother. I was supremely blessed to have not one, but two beautiful daughters.

Looking back, I wish I could have told myself the first time: "Lighten up, dummy!"

We don't get to determine how our deliveries will go, but if we are one of the lucky ones who get to do this motherhood thing, we need to strap in and do our best to enjoy the ride, however it ends up looking.

ALL ROADS LEAD TO MOTHERHOOD

Maybe none of the above applies to you—if so, you're not alone. For many women, surrogacy or adoption is preferred or necessary because it's a safer or more spiritual, practical, and/or biologically feasible way to have a child.

Finding a surrogate or an egg or sperm donor is not a process I'm equipped to advise on, but many resources and programs are available to help you navigate this world. ConceiveAbilities, a service that matches intended parents with surrogate and/or donors, also carries some book recommendations on their site.

Adoption is another great way to become a parent. Even though I know it can be overwhelming and emotionally exhausting just to find the most suitable type of adoption (domestic, international, open, private, through the foster system), my experience in this realm is also limited.

Most of what I know I owe to a wonderful memoir I read by *NYT* bestselling author Jillian Lauren called *Everything You Ever Wanted*. I also had the opportunity to interview her for my podcast, *I'm the One Pushing: A Podcast for Moms Who Live Outside the Box* (available free on iTunes), during which she elaborated on her experience of adopting her son from overseas when he was ten months old, and then, years later, adopting her second son through the foster system. Her story is a great read (or listen) for any mom.

Below is an account from yet another mom, describing meeting her now five-year-old daughter Clementine at the hospital, two hours after her birth.

> # EXCERPT FROM "WHAT TO EXPECT WHEN YOU'RE NOT EXPECTING," AS PUBLISHED IN THE *HUFFINGTON POST*
>
> **By Kathleen Dennehy of thisoldmom.com,
> Writer, Echo Park, CA, Mother of Two**
>
> "I had her."
>
> It was 4:30 p.m. I am not sentimental. But the sun actually shone brighter at that precise moment. Babymama texts me a photo of a very fresh new baby.
>
> Babymama asks me to come to her room. Thinking I'm about to meet my maybe-baby, my teeth start chattering. I'm not cold; I've just never had so much to say and no words to say it with. The baby isn't there. Babymama explains the baby is being cleaned up, because they come out with this cheese-like coating all over. "Vernix," I murmur, suddenly unable to *not* speak. "It acts as a natural moisturizer, actually good for their skin. In Europe they leave it on the babies, sometimes for days."
>
> I babble on, realizing that some women have babies and other women take classes about it.
>
> They give me a bag of clothes for the baby. Imagining Babymama and her mama shopping at Target for a child they intend to give to me breaks my heart in brand new ways I hadn't bargained for. We coo and moon over the tiny booties and Minnie Mouse T-shirts, and then I just flat out beg them to please let me see the baby. It is 6:00 p.m. and this baby has been alive for two hours and I need to imprint on someone.
>
> Babymama smiles and nods. She understands. I try not to run, but I run to the nursery to look at the baby through

a thick wall of glass. I stare at a tiny full-moon face and wonder if that face is the face of my future. I am scared that I feel nothing I can name. I try to take a picture but am told I cannot.

We ask if we can hold her. While they prepare our "bonding room," two nursing supervisors blandly ask whether we want Babymama to breastfeed the baby. I start babbling the pros and cons aloud since no social worker or adoption agency people or any one is there to advise us. Do we do what's best for the baby's health and well-being...but, by doing so, give Babymama a chance to dangerously bond and fall in love with a child that resembles no one but her? My sister, mother of four, grabs my arms and says, "You don't want her to breastfeed." We say no, full of shame.

We aren't bad people, just bad parents.

Where Should I Have My Baby?

For some women, a hospital birth is the only option due to state restrictions on home birthing and the availability of certified practitioners. This annoys me to no end, because women should be able to choose their own motherhood adventure.

Hopefully all options are available to you. I've listed them below.

A. THE HOSPITAL

Even for low-risk single pregnancies, hospitals are the top destination for most women. If you're planning (or end up having) a C-section, a hospital birth is absolutely necessary. It is also recommended if you've had any prior surgeries that could affect delivery, if you're having twins (or triplets...or octuplets, for that matter), or planning a VBAC (Vaginal Birth After C-section). In fact, it's challenging to find a midwife willing to assist with a VBAC or multiple-baby home birth.

Pushing Through the Pain

If you're certain or at least open to the idea of receiving pain medication through labor, the hospital is the only place that will dole out the heavy stuff.

The most common way to administer pain meds, or analgesics, is through an epidural. An epidural shot blocks the nerve impulses from the lower spinal segments, resulting in decreased sensation from the waist down. The local anesthetics most commonly injected through the epidural are bupivacaine, chloroprocaine, and lidocaine. They are often delivered in combination with opioids such fentanyl, morphine, or sufentanyl in order to decrease the required dose of local anesthetic.

Pain Med Dessert Menu

Epidural à la Mode

Instant relief for Mom doled out in doses through the spine, blocking pain in the appropriate area. Within safe measures, you can ask to get hit with more doses to combat the pain as you labor along.

Combined Spinal/Epidural (CSE) or Walking Epidural Soufflé

A combination of narcotics (such as fentanyl) with a lower dose of anesthesia, administered through an epidural that lasts anywhere from four to eight hours. This option supposedly allows you the freedom to walk around—hence, the name. However, that's not always feasible due to hospital policies or because it's almost as effective in numbing your lower extremities as the regular epidural.

Spinal Block Brûlée

This option is usually administered late in labor directly into the spinal-cord fluid. The anesthesia injected offers fast relief for a short period of time, but once it runs out, there's no option of continued doses as with an epidural.

Cocktail of Side Effects

Of course, any type of medication comes with the risk of side effects. But despite the cautions listed below, no long-term effects on Baby have been scientifically documented.

- Analgesics administered during birth can lower Mom's blood pressure, which can create a domino effect: contractions, labor, and Baby's heart rate may slow down as a result.

- Fewer than 1 percent of moms suffer from a severe headache and/or nausea.

- The epidural may leave a sore spot on Mom's spine that lasts for over a year. To that, I can attest.

- Some studies suggest a correlation between an epidural and having to use forceps or a vacuum to help deliver the baby. This makes sense, because while on drugs you don't feel much below your belly button, which makes it harder to push.

- Not feeling pain may also may increase Mom's risk of vaginal tearing, because she is exerting incredible strength without the ability to gauge potential damage.

- Because Baby is still connected to Mom, yes, he will take a dose of whatever analgesic is being injected. For that reason, some drugs, such as Fentanyl, are preferred over others; opioids such as Demerol, Morphine, and Butorphanol may cause short-term respiratory issues in Baby.

- Some ambiguous research correlates epidurals with latching issues.

From a study of one, the pain medication did not seem to exacerbate my wounds and had no adverse effects on my daughter's ability to breastfeed or any other negative effects after birth.

My advice: if you need the drugs, indulge guilt-free.

If you prefer, however, it's totally possible to have an unmedicated birth at the hospital.

ENJOYING A DRUG-FREE BIRTH (THE SECOND TIME AROUND)

**By Maritere Rovira Calimano,
Architect, San Juan, PR, Mother of Two**

I always thought I would get an epidural. That's until I went to a birth class and learned the pros and cons of using it.

First of all, I learned that the shot could leave long-lasting pain in my back. I also learned that pain medication can make you more likely to tear during delivery because you aren't aware when you're over-stretched. Most importantly, I didn't want my baby to be born all spaced out, having been exposed to Demerol.

At the hospital, when push came to shove—or push came to push, I should say!—my husband and my doula helped me stay the course. When I asked for an epidural during a particularly large contraction, they knew it was just the pain talking. They wiped my brow and encouraged me to push through it.

Overall, it was a nine-hour-long labor, and I pushed so hard, capillaries exploded in my cheeks and eyes. When my daughter still wouldn't come out, my husband and doctor had to manually push her down to the birth canal. On top of all of this, an episiotomy had to be performed.

I felt like I had been beaten with baseball bats.

For my second vaginal birth, I'd decided to achieve the same goal with much less pain. I had a better understanding of the birth process, and through my first experience, I had gotten to know my body better. I felt like I knew what I needed to do.

When the doctor scheduled me for an induction at 39 weeks because I was 5 mm dilated, I chose to skip the appointment. Instead, I went to an aqua-aerobics class (yeah, some people still do this).

When I finally made it to the hospital five days later on my due date, I was still at 5 mm. I was so certain I wouldn't need an epidural, I didn't even bring the extra $500 cash like I had with my first one (this was in Puerto Rico—things are done differently). They broke my water and *Boom!* I was in labor. Even though I was scared, the adrenaline and the inescapable reality of the situation helped me to focus.

My birth team was also better prepared—mentally, anyway! When we couldn't find a towel to wipe my sweat, my husband offered me a clean sock, which I used the entire time. Also, every time a contraction hit, my husband and doula each pulled up on one end of a sheet to lift my hips. We were so synchronized that I felt totally in control.

When the time came, the young *doctora* on duty let me push while kneeling, which relieves painful pressure on the back. I still don't understand the rationale of giving birth lying down. Gravity helps the baby come out!

My second daughter was born just four hours after they broke my water. This time around, I didn't feel like I had just sparred with Macho Camacho and Felix Trinidad for a world title. I was just as happy as after my first birth, but in much less pain.

Navigating the Hospital Hierarchy

At a hospital, you'll likely be assisted by your OB/GYN, a midwife, and a nurse. The delivery nurse is the real hero in most hospital birth stories; ours kicked some serious ass. The majority of hospitals also allow women to bring in doulas to assist Mom during delivery. So you *can* have your dream team at the hospital, which is important because you may need an advocate.

The truth is that the hospital staff can be induction-happy because they want to be in control of the process; it's well-documented that they're under a CYA (Cover Your Ass) insurance policy. Some also argue that hospitals want to pop moms in and out like bread in a toaster so they can put someone else in that delivery room.

The documentary film *The Business of Being Born* is a must-see for any mom-to-be. An exposé of sorts on the mainstream maternity care system in America, it had opposite its desired effect on me. Instead of persuading me to go to a birthing center or push at home, it armed me with some tools to better navigate the hospital hierarchy during labor. Of course, I don't know that I did that successfully (after reading my labor story in *Chapter 9: We Make Plans and God Laughs at Our Vaginas,* you can be the judge!), but I went to the hospital because I wanted immediate access to a full medical team and equipment should something go awry.

I also realized early on that I wasn't seeking a spiritual birth experience. Giving birth is pretty cool and all, but I didn't feel like making a "thing" out of it; I'm not much for ceremony. Laboring in a tub or being surrounded by the comforts of home didn't appeal to me as much as the safety of a clinical setting. I chose what felt right to me.

And you know what? My baby's birth still felt very intimate.

It is possible to have a beautiful birth at the hospital. But in order to do so, you may need to remind the staff that, as long as it's safe, *your* bare ass is calling the shots.

One of my major grievances was being hooked up to IVs and monitors the whole time. I wish more hospitals were encouraging of letting you roam freely around your room during labor, like the primal awesome bitch that you are. I've heard it's possible to convince the staff to leave you "untethered," but I was not successful in doing so because I was being induced.

Despite that, I did get to give birth in a warm, clean environment, in my own delivery room with a private full bathroom. I had a nice view and sunlight shining in through my window. The staff was caring (most of them) and at the end of the day I had a successful birth (alas, with the help of drugs).

Cost:

A hospital birth can cost up to $40,000 depending on where you reside, but your insurance should cover most of it. Be sure to look into your deductibles and co-pays prior to delivery so you can budget accordingly.

Also, make sure to tour the facilities before your due date. Note that most insurance providers do not cover a private room, which is too bad.

For an idea of the expenses you'll incur, please see my itemized list of charges on the next page. But before you get sticker shock, keep in mind that this was in Los Angeles. Also, it does not account for the portion paid by my insurance.

i'm the one pushing

MY HOSPITAL BILL

ACCOUNT NUMBER: ▮
DATE OF DETAIL BILL: 09/17/2015

PATIENT NAME	SEX	AGE	ADMIT DT	DISCH DT	DAYS	DT OF BIRTH
DAVILA,IVETTE GARCIA	F	36	07/12/2014	07/14/2014	2	▮

DAVILA,IVETTE GARCIA   ATTENDING PHYSICIAN: ▮

▮

INSURANCE COMPANY   GROUP NO   POLICY NO

LOS ANGELES, CA 90039

CHARGE DETAIL

SVC DT	REV CD	HCPCS	PROC CD	DESCRIPTION	QTY	CHARGES
07/12/14	0258	J7120	02580129	LACTATED RINGERS SOLP 1,00	001	383.00
07/12/14	0122		01200001	HB ROOM CHARGE 1:5 SEMI PR	001	6,778.00
07/12/14	0305	85027	03050116	HB LAB CBC HEMOGRAM W/PLT*	001	221.60
07/12/14	0300	86850	03900003	HB AB SCREEN, GEL	001	270.48
07/12/14	0300	86900	03900020	HB PATIENT ABO TYPE	001	95.82
07/12/14	0300	86901	03900023	HB PATIENT RH TYPE	001	95.82
07/13/14	0250	J2590	02502431	OXYTOCIN 250 ML BAG	002	119.00
07/13/14	0258	J7120	02580129	LACTATED RINGERS SOLP 1,00	001	383.00
07/13/14	0272		02721452	HB ANESTHESIA TRAY EPIDURA	001	960.00
07/13/14	0250	J3010	02502482	INJ, FENTANYL CITRATE, 0.1	001	60.00
07/13/14	0250		02502482	ROPIVACINE 0.2 % SOLN 100	001	60.00
07/13/14	0250		02502482	ROPIVACINE 0.2 % SOLN 100	001	60.00
07/13/14	0250		02502482	ROPIVACINE 0.2 % SOLN 100	001	60.00
07/13/14	0250	J2795	02502482	ROPIVACAINE 2 MG/ML (0.2 %	200	474.30
07/13/14	0250	J3105	02502482	TERBTLNE SULFTE UP TO 1 MG	001	60.00
07/13/14	0272		02721997	HB O2 TIME	066	166.32
07/13/14	0258	J7120	02580129	LACTATED RINGERS SOLP 1,00	001	383.00
07/13/14	0250	J2400	02502482	CHLOROPRCNE HYDRCHLRDE PER	001	80.41
07/13/14	0250	J2590	02502425	OXYTOCIN 20 UNITS/1000 ML	002	136.00
07/13/14	0250		02503101	BENZOCAINE-MENTHOL 20-0.5	001	73.30
07/13/14	0720	59409	07200015	HB VAGINAL DELIVERY	001	10,866.83
07/13/14	0710		07100054	HB RECOVERY LABOR & DELIVE	001	3,236.54
07/13/14	0272		02720332	HB IV ADMINISTRATION SET	001	297.41
07/13/14	0272		02720625	HB IV EXTENSION W/2 INJ SI	001	219.79
07/13/14	0370		03700006	HB ANES-CAT 1-BASIC OUTLYI	001	3,499.50
07/13/14	0272		02720477	HB CATHETER, FOLEY 5CC/30C	001	303.02
07/13/14	0272		02720477	HB CATHETER, FOLEY 5CC/30C	001	303.02
07/13/14	0272		02720284	HB TRAY, WITH FOLEY CATHET	001	335.09
07/13/14	0250		02503101	ERYTHROMYCIN 0.5% 5 MG/GRA	001	65.11
07/13/14	0250	J3430	02502482	INJ PHYTONDIONE (VITK) PER	001	60.00
07/13/14	0171		01710001	HB ROOM CHARGE 1:8 NSY	001	3,014.00
07/13/14	0470		04700001	HB INT NEWBORN HEARING SCR	001	439.38
07/13/14	0120		01200001	HB ROOM CHARGE 1:5 SEMI PR	001	6,778.00
07/14/14	0300	36416	03000265	HB LAB BLOOD COLLECTION FE	001	6.54
07/14/14	0309	82776	03091716	HB LAB NB GAL1PO4 URD TRAN	001	15.95
07/14/14	0309	83021	03091717	HB LAB NB HGB ELECTROPHORE	001	15.95
07/14/14	0309	84443	03090943	HB LAB NB TSH	001	15.95
07/14/14	0309	83789	03091718	HB LAB NB TANDEM MS.MS QUA	001	16.00
07/14/14	0309	83498	03091719	HB LAB NB 17-OHP	001	15.95
07/14/14	0309	82261	03090934	HB LAB BIOTINIDASE	001	15.95
07/14/14	0309	83516	03090935	HB LAB IMMUNOREACTIVE TRYP	001	15.95
07/14/14	0309	81479	03092876	HB T-CELL REC EXC CIRC (TR	001	1.00

TOTAL CHARGES   40,456.98

B. AT HOME

Home birthing is probably the most intimate way to deliver a baby. Funnily enough, assisted home births are more regulated than unassisted home births, which are legal in most states. However, I strongly advise anyone who wants to have a home birth to seek the professional assistance of a midwife and also hire a doula for the occasion. Cover your bases for the ultimate grand slam. Very few OB/GYNs will assist in a home birth, but you may be able to find one who does.

Also, you can't prepare enough for any birth, so there's no harm in mapping out the closest hospital to your home. Just in case you get beat.

There are two types of legit midwives: certified professional midwives (recognized in twenty-seven states) and certified nurse-midwives (can practice in any state). Other laws on home births and midwifery vary by state, so check with your state's licensing board to find out the restrictions in your area.

Someone very dear to me—we'll call her Esther—gave birth at home with her OB/GYN, a doula, and a midwife. Esther went into labor faster than anticipated for a first-time mom. She ended up having her baby boy on a couch covered with their shower curtain liner—props to her mom and mother-in-law who yanked it down and slid it under her in the nick of time!

Because of the speedy labor, Esther's son had crowned but her muscles weren't loosening. He was coming fast. Her OB/GYN determined that he had to perform an episiotomy so the baby could come out. An episiotomy is not something that usually happens during a home birth—but not much goes as planned in any kind of birth. In addition to the cut, Esther suffered a subsequent vaginal tear and injured her coccyx during childbirth.

What's an Episiotomy?

An episiotomy is a cut made to the superficial muscles of the perineum during labor, to widen your birth canal and help the baby exit. The incision is usually made when a speedy labor is required, if your baby is in an abnormal position, or if the perineum is not showing too much "give."

Episiotomies are often performed to prevent women from tearing during delivery, in the belief that this incision will heal more quickly than a natural tear. However, recent research suggests a cut can more easily get infected and cause complications, and can actually take longer to heal. It is also believed that cutting can lead to more severe lacerations of the anal sphincter. Therefore, while this has been a somewhat common modern procedure, some professionals are now more discerning about making the incision during an uncomplicated vaginal delivery regardless of the threat a baby's size may pose to his mom's vagina, believing that it's better to tear naturally.

Home births are best suited for women with partners who can handle this kind of labor, like Esther's partner. He was with her every step of the way. He caught the baby and cut the cord—four hours after the baby was born, as they chose to keep the baby connected to its placenta.

My husband would've fainted like a Victorian lady at the first sight of gore. But he did his best. Like Super Grover, he "showed up." He held my hand. And he avoided looking at the carnage happening in my Bermuda Triangle.

In spite of Esther's painful episiotomy *and* tear (which could've happened at the hospital), internal bruising (which could've also happened at the hospital), and tailbone injury (which could've *also* happened at the hospital), she loved having her first baby in her own home, surrounded by people she loved and trusted to fulfill her birth intentions.

Her only disappointment is that she wishes her team would've anticipated her risk of injury, so she could've tried to head it off through perineal massages.

Perineal Massage

Daily massages in the perineum starting at week 34 may increase elasticity down there, minimizing chances of a tear or episiotomy. A myriad of massage oils are marketed specifically for this purpose. If you can reach the area, you can massage it yourself; however, it may be more fun to enlist your partner and make a night of it.

Over a year later, Esther is still recovering from the physical pain her labor exerted on her and her regret over feeling she could've been better prepared. Labor wounds can be an unrelenting reminder of things gone wrong, or at least not as planned. Trauma can be quite common after birth and can be difficult to overcome.

Esther's takeaway from all of this is important to share: She found that women often minimize how they feel about their labor experience. It took Esther a while to realize that it was okay to admit what had happened, dwell on it a bit, and express to others all that she had suffered. This is part of the healing process.

Very few women get their dream anything: job, house, birth. I hope you get yours. But if you don't, support is available to help you find the tools and inner strength to overcome your grief.

Cost:

Birthing at home could save you money, depending on your insurance carrier. It's worth a call to inquire as to what all your policy covers, if anything. An assisted home birth can cost anywhere from $5,000 to $10,000 depending on your city and the fees of your labor "homies."

Birthing Woes

Birthing can be traumatic, no matter where or how you labor. It is okay to complain, cry, lick your wounds, commiserate, and most importantly, exhaust every available resource to make sure you get the answers and care you need.

The high number of women who suffer from Post Traumatic Stress Disorder (PTSD) after labor is particularly alarming. Two recent studies found that approximately one-third of all postpartum women suffer some symptoms of PTSD, and 3 to 7 percent suffer full-blown PTSD. To put this in perspective, an estimated 30 percent of Vietnam veterans have suffered PTSD in their lifetime.

Many experts have strong opinions on who's to blame, but it's worth noting that practically no women who schedule C-sections suffer from PTSD. Even women who are disappointed by unplanned C-sections and end up with a perinatal mood and anxiety disorder (PMAD) such as postpartum depression (PPD) don't seem to suffer from PTSD or have flashbacks to a traumatic birth experience.

A harrowing birth experience can be deeply scarring. Imagine lying on a table, unsure of what's happening except that strangers are sticking their hands and foreign objects inside your vagina, trying to pull out your baby and possibly mutilating you in the process—it really does sound like a horror film.

If you do have a traumatic birth experience, help is out there. Don't hesitate to get the care you need. Sharing your story with others could also lead to a better understanding and improvement of labor, delivery, and postpartum care.

c. AT A BIRTH CENTER

If you want an intimate experience away from the hospital but don't feel a home offers enough safeguards, a birth center may be the perfect fit for you.

A birth center provides a sterilized environment that is much more homey and private than a hospital. It also provides access to a professional staff of midwives, doulas, birth assistants, and registered nurses. It may also allow you to bring your own OB/GYN. Some birth centers even operate as autonomous facilities within a hospital and have affiliations with its doctors—a definite perk, in case of an emergency.

As at home, you have more freedom in a birth center than in most hospitals. You can move around the room while you endure contractions and even have the option of laboring or birthing inside a tub. They may even allow you to snack a bit before pushing!

Most birth centers don't offer epidurals, relying on other methods of pain relief such as laughing gas. You'll generally have less risk of medical intervention altogether, including resorting to a C-section. However, for a true emergency, a good birthing center will have a well-established transport-to-hospital plan.

Cost:

A birth center usually runs between $2,000 and $7,000, dependent on (a) whether your insurance provider covers this option, (b) your deductible if they do, and (c) the degree of luxury at the joint. Some high-end birth centers offer a spa-like ambiance at spa-like prices.

d. NONE OF THE ABOVE

Babies wait for no one, and you may end up delivering your baby in the car, in an elevator, or at the grocery store. My mom's water broke at checkout—*after* she paid, a fact she never ceases to highlight when she tells the story. She made it to the hospital, but what if she hadn't? I could've been born at Pueblo, a now-defunct supermarket chain in Puerto Rico.

Signs of Labor

Labor happens differently to all of us, but for a first-time mom, it's hard to know if it's really about to happen. The telltale signs can be misleading because the contractions can be either too faint or too strong. However, there are a few things that do happen before one pops that baby out.

Lightening

Baby drops lower into the pelvis in preparation for birth—ideally, head first. When this occurs, Baby may feel lighter on your diaphragm but heavier on your bladder.

Bloody Show

As gross as it sounds, this pink or brownish discharge indicates that the mucous plug has "retired," opening the cervix for showbiz. This is an indication that your cervix has completely effaced (refer to "SAT-Worthy Labor Vocabulary" in the next chapter, for a definition).

Contractions, Real Ones

Well, *all* contractions are real, but Mom's uterus contracts during her entire pregnancy in preparation for childbirth, so how do you know when they are *the* ones? Labor contractions start in the back, like a dull pain, and move their way towards the front. They escalate into very painful cramps (sometimes you may even feel them in your anus) and appear at regular intervals.

Contractions that indicate labor last from 30 to 90 seconds and won't go away by changing positions or shouting a mantra. They're truly relentless until you give birth. It's recommended you wait until they become acute and regular: four to five minutes apart for at *least* two hours. To measure contractions, you need to set the timer from the start of one contraction to the start of the following one.

Waterworks

Commonly known as your "water breaking." The protective sac filled with amniotic fluid surrounding Baby will likely pop at some point, or it may have to be ruptured prior to labor. Moms may leak fluid for days prior to delivery, or the sac may burst like a water balloon at an inopportune moment. We're at its mercy.

It's important to let your doctor or midwife know if you're leaking amniotic fluid to prevent Baby from getting an infection.

I had been planning to search for a powerful yet unexpected birth story to share with you, when suddenly the narrative plopped into my inbox, like a bundled baby dropped off by a stork. One of the hundreds of moms I once interviewed for a TV pilot, a Minnesotean mother of six, shared her son's Facebook post with me about his wife, Alex. Her extraordinary birth story didn't go exactly as planned.

But it *did* go exactly as it should've.

BACKSEAT BABY

**By Alex Elliott,
Howell, MI, Piano Teacher, Mother of Five**

After making it through four pregnancies in five years, my husband and I were pretty set with two boys and two girls. I had worked hard to lose all of my baby weight and had purged our home of baby items and maternity clothes. But what a wonderful surprise to find out we were expecting baby number five! I was determined to make this last pregnancy and labor my best one yet.

I read natural childbirthing books and discovered ways to work with my body and enjoy my labor. We chose to have the baby with a midwife at an alternative birthing center set up inside a local hospital.

Near the end of my pregnancy, I calculated that Friday would be the exact same day of my pregnancy that both of my other girls had been born—38 weeks and 1 day—so I went to bed Thursday night pretty much expecting to go into labor. I had also gotten acupuncture a few days prior, to help bring it on. Our house was ready for our little girl to arrive, and my hospital bag was almost packed.

At about 3:00 a.m. I woke to a contraction that was pretty strong but still not painful. I laid in bed for the next hour and started tracking the contractions on an app on my phone. They came about every ten minutes or so for the next hour, so I decided to get up and finish packing my hospital bag. As soon as I got up and moved around, the contractions started coming faster, about three to four minutes apart, but they were not as strong or long as the ones I had been having in bed. Confused, I laid back down and tracked them for another hour; they went back to being about ten minutes apart and consistently stronger. I woke up my husband and told him it was time to go.

I quickly put on mascara and called my midwife to let her know we were heading in. The contractions were now coming more intensely. My previous labors had ranged from ninety minutes to about six hours, and this felt like a fast one!

While waiting for my husband, I started the van and scraped the snow and ice off the windows. My labor was picking up so much, I knew we'd have to rush to make it the hospital!

I had been having contractions for almost three hours as we got on our way. I sat in the back seat directly behind my husband; I didn't want to sit in front because I needed room to move with the contractions, and there were car seats in the other two back spots.

I had been preparing myself throughout this pregnancy to have a joyful labor that was completely free of fear. So with each contraction, I was smiling and sometimes even laughing; I was honestly enjoying the process of working with my body to open up and have this baby. I wasn't afraid of the pain, so it almost didn't feel like pain at all! Pain is a psychological response to feeling unsafe. Your brain registers pain to alert you that something is wrong, but childbirth is completely natural—it's not usually unsafe or wrong.

The contractions took some intense focus and concentration to get through, but it was totally manageable for me. I'm sure it being my fifth baby helped. I knew what was happening.

Between contractions, I texted our mothers to let them know we were on our way to the hospital and called my midwife again to let her know things were really picking up. I even updated my Facebook status! But I must have sounded *too* relaxed and calm on the phone with my midwife, because she assumed she still had some time.

As we neared the hospital, a car cut us off, causing us to miss our exit off the highway. So we had to get off at the next exit and drive through a subdivision to get to the hospital.

I was now at the point where I needed to groan with the contractions to help me get through them. As we drove past the houses, I felt a big contraction with the urge to push, and my water broke! I knew that meant the baby was coming out with the next contraction. I turned around in my seat to face the back because I had read that pushing a baby out on all fours was the best position for giving birth.

Meanwhile, my husband had no idea what was going on. He was on the phone with his boss telling him that he wasn't coming in to work that day. And I was so focused on my labor that I didn't have time to update him!

Sure enough, the next contraction pushed the baby's head out. I consciously relaxed to let it come out slowly enough that I wouldn't tear. Then I immediately yanked my sweatpants to my knees and yelled "Pull over!"

My husband pulled to the side of the road in the subdivision, about two minutes away from the hospital. He got out and opened the sliding door of the van and was shocked to see our little girl's head already out! I asked him if he could help pull her out, but then another contraction came and I told him to just catch her! The rest of her slipped right out and into my husband's hands.

When my husband caught her, he let out a laugh of pure joy. I will never forget that sound. The cord was around her neck, so he unwrapped it, and then she made some noise and started to cry a little. Meanwhile, a group of morning joggers passed by across the street, totally oblivious to what was happening with us!

I was still on all fours with my sweatpants at my knees, and my pants had caught almost all of the mess of giving birth, which was great for the car! The cord was still attached to both me and the baby, so my husband had to pass our daughter through my legs so I could grab her and turn around to sit and hold her. It was snowing outside, but I was wearing a big comfy sweatshirt; I covered her as best as I could with my big sleeves. My little baby girl was so content all snuggled in with me, and I was happy to be finally holding her!

My husband got back in the front and drove the rest of the short way to the hospital. When we pulled into the emergency entrance area, my husband went in to get help. I don't think he was very clear as to what had happened, because everyone seemed confused and didn't know what to do. A security guard came over with a wheelchair and opened the door to see me sitting in the seat with a newborn baby, cord still attached, and an awful mess in my pants! He quickly realized that a wheelchair wasn't going to cut it, so he closed the door again to keep the cold air out of the car.

Finally a crew came back out with a stretcher and I was able to get my pants and shoes off and get in the bed. As they wheeled me into the emergency room, they all seemed to be in shock! It was like they couldn't comprehend what they were seeing because I was just sitting comfortably, smiling and holding a baby that was also content. I think it messed with them to see us so calm and relaxed.

Once inside, a crowd of hospital staff just stood around staring at us. Finally, one of the emergency room doctors checked me to make sure everything looked good and they cut the cord. They wanted to start an IV in me, but I refused since there was no apparent reason that I needed one.

My midwife arrived to deliver the placenta and then she took us to our room. We cleaned up a little bit and I got in a hospital gown while they weighed the baby and wrapped her in some clean blankets. She was 6 pounds even.

We spent the next day resting and enjoying our new baby girl. The whole experience was beautiful, and I wouldn't have had it any other way!

TO EACH HER OWN

It is likely (pending an impromptu labor in a minivan, like Alex) that you'll be able to choose where you labor. And it is our right as "pushers" to fight for our desired experiences.

However, to *push it* onto others is crossing a line.

One person's idea of a romantic weekend could involve walking blindfolded into a path of fresh rose petals that leads to a candle-lit bed and culminates in tantric sex to the beat of Sade. She may prefer to birth at home or at a birth center.

I'm the kind of gal who wants to be fucked hard and fast against a cold glass sliding door for all of three minutes and then pass out watching *Law and Order: SVU.* I have, on most days, a non-romantic, practical approach to sex. I had a similar approach to labor. That's why I chose a hospital.

But for some, birthing at a hospital is reneging on woman-ity. For others, birthing any other place is irresponsible. Can we unite in motherhood instead of divide?

Crack houses excluded, there's no right or wrong place to labor. We're all trying to reach the same goal: a healthy mama and baby.

THE MORAL OF YOUR BIRTH STORY

For better or worse, a regular pregnancy lasts a little over nine months. We can use this time to look both inward and outward.

Studying other women's birth stories can help us accept unpredictability, as well as imagine what we would do if A, B, or C were to happen.

Plan to labor in a place that feels safe, wherever that may be. If you have others who are planning on being in the room, make sure they are all on your same page regarding birth intentions. If they know what Mom wants, they can help advocate if there's pressure in the room to do something that doesn't feel right.

Also, hand-picking the professionals who will assist in the delivery can help immensely—whether it's a doula, a nurse, a midwife, and/or an OB/GYN. You've got to trust your entourage.

But understand that even having done your due diligence and with your fantasy team on your side, some circumstances will be out of your control. You may have to make fast choices. This will be hard. Particularly if your choices are influenced by fear: fear of something going fatally wrong, of your instincts betraying you, of being led astray by your caregivers, and most importantly, that you'll regret your final chess move. Fear is not your friend; try not to let it take over your experience. If you must change course due to circumstances out of your control, try to remember that your mind can be as bendy as your body. Let it open up, too.

Of course, it is wise to be wary of anyone trying to change your birth plan intentions without a sound medical reason. But conversely, there's nothing wrong with having a little faith in modern medicine and technology. Not every doctor has a secret agenda to cut you open and rip the baby from your womb so they can go on a fishing trip. A compassionate and knowledgeable OB/GYN will always have Mom's—and Baby's—best interest at heart.

And most importantly, trust your womb.

It'll get you there.

To Doula or Not to Doula?

The word "doula" comes from the Greek word *doulos*, which means "slave." However, DONA International (Doulas of North America), sugarcoats it a bit by translating it as "women who serve." Both meanings are correct, etymologically speaking.

A doula's purpose is to assist a woman throughout her pregnancy, during childbirth, and post-natally. In spite of (most likely) not having a medical degree, a doula brings emotional and physical wisdom to a mom before, during, and after birth. A good doula is empowering, nurturing, knowledgeable, and connected with the process of childbirth. She (or he) is unafraid to be in the line of fire during your delivery.

A doula often has a more intimate approach to childbirth than a doctor. A labor doctor can be like a successful actor who comes to Academy Awards just to give the Oscar to the next in line and then "peaces out" (a la Leonardo DiCaprio). He's only going to be in the room during the highlights of your delivery. Some doctors come in just to catch the baby.

Requirements for doula-hood vary from institution to institution, but generally speaking, to become a Certified Labor Doula (CLD), one must attend a certain number of births, receive a particular number of recommendations, study and/or attend workshops on birth, breastfeeding, and postpartum care, and pass program- and course-specific trainings and assessments.

These days, finding a doula is easy...but finding *the* doula is harder. Type "doula" in any search engine and you'll get a long list of websites that will help you find doulas in your area. There's even an online matchmaking service, DoulaMatch.net, which connects you with doulas all over the U.S. and Canada, verifying qualifications and providing testimonials from other families.

To determine the right doula for you, you may want to cross-check the doula's references and credentials, talk to previous clients, and have an in-person interview to see if you have good chemistry; you will be spending a lot of time with this person. Also, make sure you go over what's expected. I recently interviewed a mom for my podcast who was quite disappointed because her doula didn't massage her during her long labor. By the time her doula was ready to dole out the goods, my friend was too close to delivery and in too much in pain to want to be touched.

Prior to becoming pregnant, I was certain I would hire a doula. Why? Because I'm married to a man who wished we lived in the seventies just so he could pace the hospital hallways with a cigar between his lips while I pushed our baby. The thought of having an experienced labor veteran with a soothing voice and massaging hands next to me was very appealing.

A doula cannot only help determine when it's time to push, be an advocate in a hospital room, and prevent unnecessary procedures, including an unwanted C-section, but she can help you adjust to life with a newborn. She can support you through breastfeeding. She can at times feel like your best friend.

In the end, that was a problem for me. My husband and I didn't want to share our intimate birth moments with any invested third party—including our relatives. We welcomed the clinical demeanor of the hospital staff. Don't get me wrong: I never felt unassisted, unheard, or unsupported; I just didn't feel overindulged. Which can be wonderful and may be exactly what *you* want!

The majority of my friends who did hire a doula were happy with their experience, too. A great doula is an asset. If you want an ally to help you deliver your baby, start now in finding your *doulmate*.

Do I Bank That Cord?

If cord blood banking were free, everyone would take precautionary measures to safe-keep their child's stem cells. But like many other birth-related services, private cord blood banks are a business. They have aggressive marketing campaigns and some say they prey on the fear of vulnerable parents. And it ain't cheap. Collection ranges from $1,000 to $2,500 and storage ranges from $100 to $300 per year.

The truth is that storing a newborn's umbilical cord provides an abundant pool of stem cells that could potentially treat different forms of leukemia, lymphoma, and anemia. If your family has a history of any of these conditions, you may want to consider banking your baby's cord, as it could save not only your baby's life but the life of any family members who are a match. (Siblings have a 25 percent chance of being a perfect match.) Some private banks will even give you a discount to collect and/or store cord blood if you provide appropriate documentation of relevant family medical history.

Moreover, additional cord blood benefits could possibly surface in coming years. Researchers are studying other ways the cells could be useful; for example, in treating cerebral palsy and autism.

However, according to the American Society for Blood and Marrow Transplantation, the chance of a healthy person needing her own stem cells are only .04 percent. Therefore, most experts agree that the best option is to donate your child's cord blood to a public bank, as it's free and many others outside your family could be a match and benefit from these rich cells.

Furthermore, if your child were to need stem cells further down the line, chances are that her own blood cells collected at birth would have the same disease she's hoping to fight.

Therefore, banking privately is like purchasing travel insurance: You'll probably never need it and if you do, it probably won't cover you, though you'd be so happy if it does.

Taking all that into consideration, in short(ish): If there's no medical history pointing to it, the likelihood of your needing your baby's cord is (thankfully) next to none, and if you were to need it (unfortunately) it may not help you, but it could (fortunately) help a relative or even a stranger. You can always also discard it, but why waste perfectly amazing cells that could save someone's life?

My advice? If you have the money and/or a specific medical reason, bank that cord. If you don't, bank it publicly. You can arrange this with your hospital or inquire about mail-in programs at the Parent's Guide to Cord Blood Foundation (www.parentsguidetocordblood.org).

I would've practiced what I'm preaching and gone with the public bank, but my husband and mother-in-law felt very strongly that we go private. We chose Cord Blood Bank and it was so easy—they send you a kit that you bring to the hospital. Once the baby is born, the nurse takes the blood and tissue needed, puts it in the box, and the bank makes sure it reaches its climate-controlled destination. Somewhere, my baby's cord blood lives in a cooler.

Do I Keep Baby Connected to the Mother "Landline"?

Yet another choice we must face is whether or not to cut the umbilical cord right away or leave Baby connected to the placenta after birth. Referred to as "placental transfusion," this process allows the transfer of oxygen-rich blood to flow into the infant, increasing hemoglobin levels.

Traditionally, it was believed that waiting to cut the cord could lead to excessive blood loss in Mom and increase birth complications and the risk of jaundice in Baby. However, current research indicates that delaying cutting the cord does not pose any threats to either Mom or Baby. In fact, it can be quite beneficial.

According to studies, a prolonged contact with the placenta after birth may help increase iron stores in infants, reducing risk of anemia. A recent analysis also found that waiting a little over three minutes to cut the cord could improve fine motor and social skills. There's even a school of thought that encourages mothers to keep their babies attached to their placenta for days. Look up "Lotus Births" to learn more.

For preterm infants (born before thirty-seven weeks), delayed cord clamping can be a game-changer. It improves red blood cell volume and circulation. Studies also show that it decreases the risk of brain hemorrhage and necrotizing enterocolitis, a serious intestinal disease.

However, delayed cord clamping is not always recommended. If an emergency arises, such as Baby being unable to breathe, the cord needs to be cut immediately.

The general recommendations from authorities vary: The WHO and APA say the cord should be clamped within the first minute; the American College of Nurse-Midwives suggest to wait five minutes for full-term infants if Baby is placed skin-on-skin on Mama's chest, or two minutes if Baby is at or below the height of the birth canal.

I had planned on waiting, but my birth story wrote itself.

WTF Is Apgar?

When you give birth at a hospital, nurses perform tests to rate the health level of the following five items. While the tests are so named for their creator, anesthesiologist Virginia Apgar, they are sometimes listed to create an acronym:

- **A**ppearance (skin color)

- **P**ulse (heart rate)

- **G**rimace response (reflexes)

- **A**ctivity (and muscle tone)

- **R**espiration (breathing)

Apgar tests are usually done twice: one minute after birth and again five minutes after birth. The overall score ranges from zero to ten. A baby who scores seven or higher is considered very healthy. But a lower score doesn't always mean something is wrong. Perfectly healthy babies often have low Apgar scores in the first minute of life. In more than 98 percent of cases, the Apgar score reaches seven after five minutes of life. When it does not, the baby needs close monitoring and perhaps even medical care.

Placenta Smoothie, Por Favor

Placentophagy is the act of mammals eating the placenta of their offspring after they are born. Some experts believe placentophagy stemmed from a survival instinct: as a way for a mother to hide any evidence of her tender baby so that predators would steer clear—not as a form of supplemental nourishment.

In modern times, human placentophagy has become a headline. Celebrities are seen making smoothies out of their placenta or having it encapsulated to take as supplements after delivery.

Placenta-eating advocates claim that consuming their own nutrient-rich placentas helps moms boost milk supply and avoid postpartum depression. Yet, the evidence is at best anecdotal and the benefits cited could very well have been a placebo effect.

Although many women have ingested their placentas to no harm, the CDC recently issued a warning advising against this practice, after a baby was hospitalized with GBS. Although other factors couldn't be ruled out, the bacteria was determined to have come from the placenta capsules, which tested positive for the same strain of bacteria.

Some women have reported feeling over-stimulated by it, with sensations similar to drinking too much caffeine, while others have listed headaches and excessive burping as side effects.

My friend Claire swears by it, though, saying ingesting her placenta in a series of pills and smoothies made her feel like she had an acute sensorial set of superpowers. I look up to her, so her word is good in my book. And yet—I wasn't curious enough to shell out the $300 to get someone to juice my placenta.

If you are interested in placenta consumption, seek an experienced "encapsulator" with a bloodborne pathogen certification and a dedicated lab, not a home kitchen

Do I Give Baby Erythromycin?

This is the gooey Vaseline-like substance they put on your baby's eyes, gluing them shut for a few days. The medical definition of erythromycin is "an antibiotic cream used preventatively to keep a baby from contracting olphthalmia neonatorum (ON), a type of pink eye that could cause blindness." Before you freak out, know that this disease is treatable with antibiotics and blindness is highly unlikely.

Babies are only exposed to this viral or bacterial infection if Mom has herpes, gonorrhea, or chlamydia. If that's the case, erythromycin is necessary because Baby's eyes may become infected during vaginal birth. It's improbable for a baby born via C-section to contract ON.

Although I'm STD-free, we went with the flow and let the nurses administer erythromycin. The cream is harmless, but the negative is that Baby's eyes are then shut, which may cause her further confusion about her new surroundings and delay her bonding with parents.

"She was so alert," complained my husband, "and then they put that shit on her eyes and I lost her for the next few days."

If there's a next baby, we may skip the erythromycin—*if* our state allows, that is. Most hospitals are required by law to apply the ointment.

Vitamin K…Krazy or Kool?

Vitamin K aids in the coagulation of blood. Newborns are born deficient in this vitamin, regardless of maternal intake, because it doesn't easily cross the placenta. Vitamin K also doesn't transfer into breast milk, so most babies who experience a deficiency are exclusively breastfed. Babies don't build an appropriate store of this vitamin until they extract it from solids.

The danger of a vitamin K deficiency is that a baby may develop uncontrolled bleeding in the brain and/or the intestines. Although rare, this can occur within hours or up to twenty-four weeks of being born. Undiagnosed, this bleeding can have severe effects, including loss of gross motor skills, developmental issues, organ failure, and even death.

A vitamin K shot can prevent all this. The APA recommends to administer it intramuscularly soon after birth. As always, though, there are concerns. Critics argue that the injected substance is synthetic, is too high a dosage for an infant's liver to handle, and contains questionable ingredients, most notably the disputed propylene glycol (rated as "low" hazard by the Environmental Working Group). Many also quote a study linking vitamin K shots to leukemia; however, that study has been debunked repeatedly by larger and more thorough analyses.

The most serious side effect ever documented—and it's serious—is the case of a newborn suffering anaphylactic shock (which thankfully wasn't fatal). The only other cited consequence has been bruising at the injection site.

Given this dearth of negative outcomes, the benefits of the shot seem to outweigh the risks. Statistics show that the odds of internal bleeding going unnoticed are higher than any negative reaction to being pricked—and the consequences of the oversight being exponentially higher. However, if the injection gives you the heebie-jeebies, you can opt out of it, or you can ask for an oral dose of vitamin K to be administered, though it is believed to be less effective.

Circumspect About Circumcision?

Circumcision is an elective surgical procedure that removes the foreskin of the penis, exposing the top of it. In adulthood, circumcision makes a penis look like Darth Vader: the head looks like the little helmet and the shaft looks like the cape. A friend of mine masterfully likened an uncircumcised penis to Oakleys stuffed inside their sunglass bag.

A circumcision is usually performed during the first ten days of life, commonly even forty-eight hours after baby's birth. For many parents, circumcision is a no-brainer; this practice is often based on cultural and religious principles. But it can be an agonizing dilemma for parents who don't ascribe to any traditions that embrace or reject circumcision. A choice of "yes" is irreversible, after all. Once circumcised, never uncircumcised again.

Some of the cited perks of being circumcised are suffering fewer urinary tract infections, having a lower risk of penile cancer, and for heterosexual men, having a decreased chance of contracting HIV or an STD. However, many HIV findings come from studies in areas with a high incidence of HIV; some experts agree that they can't be applied to the less HIV-ridden population of the U.S.

Most people agree that it's easier to keep a circumcised penis clean and this prevents infection, inflammation, and irritation. Those who disagree argue that circumcision can heighten the chance of infection, especially during diaper-wearing years when the penis is exposed to whatever comes out of its smelly neighbor in the rear.

Other known risks of circumcision include complications during the procedure such as infection, abnormal bleeding, and urinary problems. Not to mention the pain that Baby undergoes. Cosmetically speaking, I've also heard of "botched" penis jobs.

Parents who choose not to circumcise often cite that they don't want their son to suffer unnecessary pain. They also may feel wary of the anesthesia given during the procedure. This is usually administered in the form of either a topical cream, a suppository, or an injectable.

Lastly, some parents feel that it's not their right to decide on their son's behalf, so they leave it untouched until their son is old enough to choose on his own between the "Darth Vader" and the "Oakley bag."

Ultimately, the American Academy of Pediatrics states that the health benefits of circumcision outweigh the risks, but that at the same time, there isn't enough sound evidence to recommend circumcision for all newborn boys. In short: they're not for it or against it. So it's all up to the parents.

And it's not a decision to be taken lightly.

If you do choose to circumcise, make sure to go over the procedure and form of anesthesia with your doctor to make sure you make an informed decision that is right for your family. The healing may take up to ten days.

If you choose not to circumcise, wash the area very carefully with warm water. But in the beginning, do *not* pull back the foreskin to clean beneath it. After a while, the foreskin can be gently pulled away until resistance is met. Full retraction of the foreskin may not happen until a boy is three years or older.

So...do you know if you're circumcising? Or still circumspect about the whole thing?

Map Your Own Adventure

Labor and Delivery (L&D) is a choose-your-own-adventure experience, written by your body, fate, labor helpers, and your child's will. You'll get to make a few calls as the story unfolds. But unlike a choose-your-own-adventure, you can't reverse or recant your decisions. You'll never know what would've happened.

You'll only know what turns you took and where you landed.

Because my choices felt so overwhelming, I made a map that helped me see all the options laid out. It's in the next spread and I've also included it at the front of this book for easy reference. I hope it helps you trek your own track—as much as the stars allow.

Happy travels!

My Birth

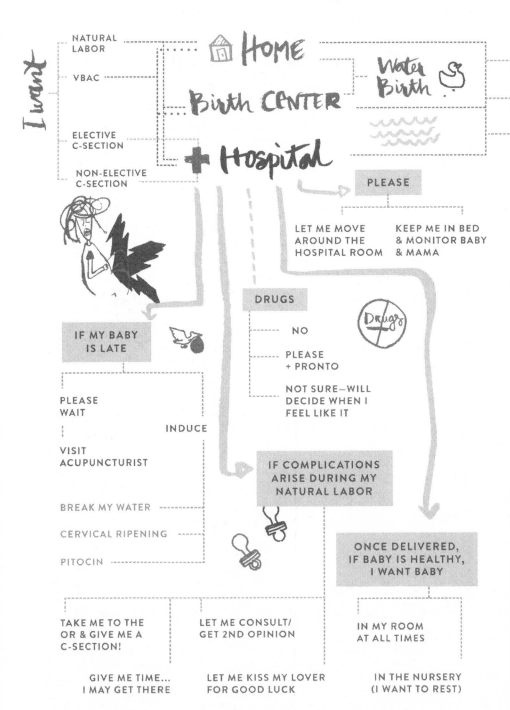

I want

NATURAL LABOR ········
VBAC ········
ELECTIVE C-SECTION ········
NON-ELECTIVE C-SECTION ········

🏠 Home
Birth CENTER
✚ Hospital

Water Birth 🦆

PLEASE

LET ME MOVE AROUND THE HOSPITAL ROOM

KEEP ME IN BED & MONITOR BABY & MAMA

IF MY BABY IS LATE

PLEASE WAIT

VISIT ACUPUNCTURIST

INDUCE

BREAK MY WATER

CERVICAL RIPENING

PITOCIN

DRUGS

NO

PLEASE + PRONTO

NOT SURE—WILL DECIDE WHEN I FEEL LIKE IT

Drugs

IF COMPLICATIONS ARISE DURING MY NATURAL LABOR

ONCE DELIVERED, IF BABY IS HEALTHY, I WANT BABY

TAKE ME TO THE OR & GIVE ME A C-SECTION!

LET ME CONSULT/ GET 2ND OPINION

IN MY ROOM AT ALL TIMES

GIVE ME TIME... I MAY GET THERE

LET ME KISS MY LOVER FOR GOOD LUCK

IN THE NURSERY (I WANT TO REST)

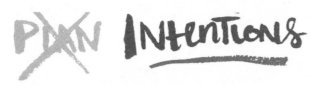

PAIN INTENTIONS

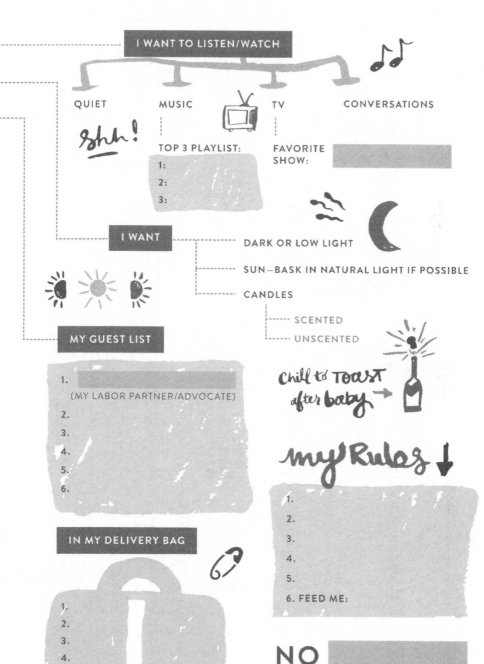

I WANT TO LISTEN/WATCH

QUIET   MUSIC   TV   CONVERSATIONS

Shh!

TOP 3 PLAYLIST:

1:

2:

3:

FAVORITE SHOW:

I WANT

DARK OR LOW LIGHT

SUN—BASK IN NATURAL LIGHT IF POSSIBLE

CANDLES

SCENTED

UNSCENTED

Chill to TOAST after baby →

MY GUEST LIST

1.
(MY LABOR PARTNER/ADVOCATE)

2.

3.

4.

5.

6.

my Rules ↓

1.

2.

3.

4.

5.

6. FEED ME:

IN MY DELIVERY BAG

1.

2.

3.

4.

5.

NO

ALLOWED, PLEASE!

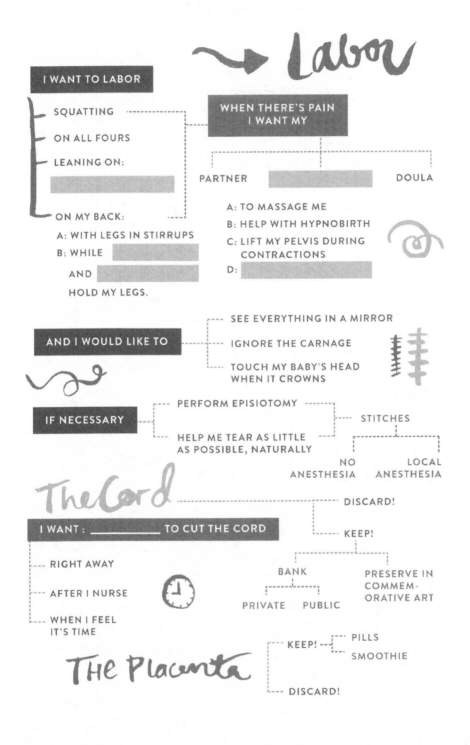

Labor

I WANT TO LABOR

- SQUATTING
- ON ALL FOURS
- LEANING ON:
- ON MY BACK:
  - A: WITH LEGS IN STIRRUPS
  - B: WHILE
    AND
    HOLD MY LEGS.

WHEN THERE'S PAIN I WANT MY

PARTNER   DOULA

- A: TO MASSAGE ME
- B: HELP WITH HYPNOBIRTH
- C: LIFT MY PELVIS DURING CONTRACTIONS
- D:

AND I WOULD LIKE TO

- SEE EVERYTHING IN A MIRROR
- IGNORE THE CARNAGE
- TOUCH MY BABY'S HEAD WHEN IT CROWNS

IF NECESSARY

- PERFORM EPISIOTOMY
- HELP ME TEAR AS LITTLE AS POSSIBLE, NATURALLY

STITCHES

NO ANESTHESIA   LOCAL ANESTHESIA

The Cord

DISCARD!

KEEP!

I WANT : _____ TO CUT THE CORD

- RIGHT AWAY
- AFTER I NURSE
- WHEN I FEEL IT'S TIME

BANK

PRIVATE   PUBLIC

PRESERVE IN COMMEM-ORATIVE ART

THE Placenta

KEEP! -- PILLS
        SMOOTHIE

DISCARD!

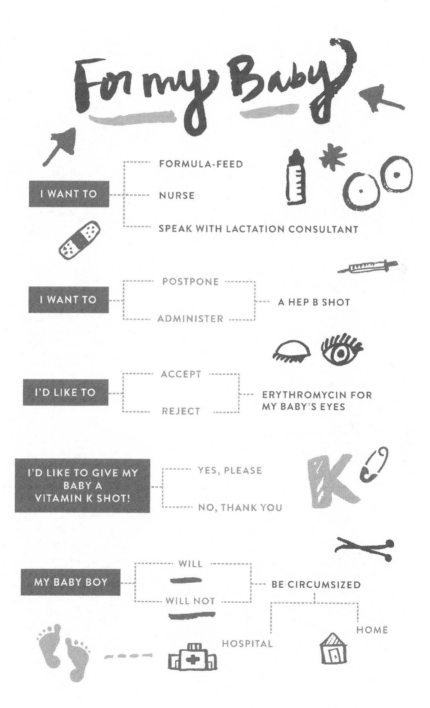

For my Baby

I WANT TO
- FORMULA-FEED
- NURSE
- SPEAK WITH LACTATION CONSULTANT

I WANT TO
- POSTPONE
- ADMINISTER
→ A HEP B SHOT

I'D LIKE TO
- ACCEPT
- REJECT
→ ERYTHROMYCIN FOR MY BABY'S EYES

I'D LIKE TO GIVE MY BABY A VITAMIN K SHOT!
- YES, PLEASE
- NO, THANK YOU

MY BABY BOY
- WILL
- WILL NOT
→ BE CIRCUMSIZED
- HOSPITAL
- HOME

WE MAKE PLANS AND GOD LAUGHS AT OUR VAGINAS

My Birthing Story: A Page-One Rewrite

I HAD CAREFULLY OUTLINED my daughter's birth story. Here's the gist of what I wanted: (1) to wait it out for the big, clock-timed contractions at home, (2) to have a drug-free and untethered vaginal birth at the hospital, and (3) to keep my baby connected to the placenta for the first minutes of her life while I nursed her. I knew that I had to leave a little wiggle room to fate, but I was pretty certain I could achieve what I felt to be my pretty reasonable birth plan.

But as it turned out, I had to shove the whole thing through the shredder.

"You Can't Always Get What You Want"

One week past my due date, my husband and I sat in my OB/GYN's office to review our options. I was at the end of week 40 and my cervix showed no signs of dilation—or so I was told.

The doctor explained our situation: My baby was already eight pounds and my placenta was calcifying—which means dying. Foreboding, yes, but placental calcification is expected; the placenta was not meant to last much longer than nine months.

The real problem was, my baby also ran the risk of meconium aspiration. *WTF is meconium?* I wondered. I imagined it to be a brew of congealed stools, chewing tobacco spit, sidewalk-peeled gum, unmenstruated blood, nine months of unborn baby snot, and what's left of Steven Segal's hair.

Doctors, however, say meconium is the earliest bowel movement of your baby—a tar-like smoothie of epithelial cells (tissue that lines up glands and stuff), lanugo (baby's fur, much like Segal's), mucus (I was partially right!), amniotic fluid, bile, and water. Simply put, it's shit. Like we need more of that.

The concern is that when you're overdue, your now fully developed baby may poop in your womb and eat it. Or, most accurately, gasp it. If so, chances are she'll be just fine; Los Angeles' air pollution is probably worse. However, there's a slight chance that inhaled meconium combined with amniotic fluid could partially or completely block your baby's airways. This is known as Meconium Aspiration Syndrome (MAS), and many newborns spend time in the Neonatal Intensive Care Unit (NICU) because of it. The more shit baby breathes, the more serious MAS can be. It can cause chemical irritation to the lung tissue, airway obstruction, infection, and/or inhibition of the lung's capacity to properly expand.

So when the doctor told us all this, I had some questions. And I've never been much for beating around the bush. Especially when it's *my* bush.

```
                IVETTE
        So let me get this straight:
        My placenta is about to
        expire, our already big baby
        could get even bigger in
        utero, giving me a vaganus
        when pushed out, after
        eating her own shit, which
```

```
could lead to a serious
condition that might send
her to the NICU?

        DOCTOR
Pretty much.
```

I was angry. Induced labor was *not* supposed to be on the menu.

I'd once read that Eskimo women pop a squat, dig a hole in the snow, push out their baby, and cut the umbilical cord with their teeth. Russian peasants, I'd heard, used to step away from the job line, deliver their baby in an open field, put it in a sling, and then go back to harvesting potatoes or whatever they were yielding to make more vodka—cuz who doesn't need a shot of it after that?

Why on earth couldn't I push my baby the way I had envisioned it? I leaned in closer, almost perched on top of my OB/GYN's desk, face-to-face with his Golden Uterus Award.

```
        IVETTE
Will I have to take Pitocin?

        DOCTOR
Yes.

        IVETTE
Isn't Pitocin bad for the
baby? Won't it lead to a
(gasp!) C-section?
```

I hated saying the C-word out loud. Like many other twats, I thought I was above the cut. I was also terrified of Pitocin: the "gateway drug," as some refer to it. I had heard that Pitocin contractions are hard on the baby and that they are so painful you inevitably need an epidural (which I didn't want), which in turn often leads to a Level 4 tear (which I definitely didn't want) because you don't feel your vagina ripping in half during the pushing part. And in some cases, you may end up with a C-section (which I really, really, *really* didn't want).

Needless to say, I wanted to avoid Pitocin at all costs.

The Lowdown on Pitocin

Just as folic acid is to folate, Pitocin is the synthetic form of oxytocin—a hormone released during labor that causes contractions. Pitocin basically poses as oxytocin in order to make your uterus contract.

Pitocin's package insert lists its risks: fetal heart abnormalities (slow heartbeat, PVCs, and arrhythmias), low Apgar scores (see previous chapter for an explanation), neonatal jaundice, neonatal retinal hemorrhage, permanent central nervous system or brain damage, and fetal death. Potential risks for Mom are water intoxication, pulmonary edema, and abnormal sodium levels.

Some claim that Pitocin increases the risk of a C-section almost twofold; but with so many variables, it's hard to pinpoint whether or not the eventual need for a C-section was a direct consequence of Pitocin. However, it is a fact that the use of Pitocin doesn't lower C-section rates.

In spite of its bad rep and the warning signs on the packet, a 2011 Cochrane Review concluded that Pitocin "did not seem to harm mothers or babies and appeared to shorten labor times by nearly two hours."

Our OB/GYN, referred to by the hospital staff as "The *BEST*," patiently demystified our hearsay concerns.

                    DOCTOR
          Some women think Pitocin
          intensifies labor pain
          because they weren't feeling

```
any labor pain before they
took the drug. Labor hurts.
It's supposed to hurt.
```

```
            IVETTE
      (under breath)
No shit, Sherlock.
```

Acclaimed OB/GYN and author Jennifer Ashton, M.D., agrees with my doc: "As an obstetrician AND a mom who has [had] two babies (one with and one without Pitocin), I did not experience any difference in my two labor experiences. However, every woman is different, and every woman is entitled to her own subjective experience and opinions thereof" ("Study Raises Concern Pitocin May Harm Babies," ABC News, May 10, 2013).

But I refused to throw in the towel. My husband held his breath, hoping I would just agree to go with the flow. *Does he not know me after fifteen years?!*

```
            IVETTE
Isn't there something else I
can do?

            DOCTOR
      (not hopeful)
We could try to induce
with Cytotec or vaginal
misoprostol for cervical
ripening.
```

Cervical ripening? WTF? I imagined Fabio on a horse tearing through a giant vagina. The erotic novel cover I was visualizing was interrupted by the real explanation.

> DOCTOR
> A low dose of Vaginal
> Misoprostol could help
> speed things along without
> significant differences in
> C-section rates or fetal
> outcomes.

I felt like Keanu in *The Matrix.* Red pill or blue? Pitocin or Vaginal Misoprowhatever?

I chose the intravaginal pill and hoped it would ripen my cervix (Eww!) so I could have this baby *almost* as planned.

Much later, I found out that Cytotec was actually created to prevent peptic ulcers but is frequently used off-label in obstetrics to prompt labor, because it helps the cervix dilate. However, it is not recommended for use on pregnant women by the U.S. FDA, the WHO, and pretty much every obstetric organization in the world except the American College of Obstetricians and Gynecologists, because it may cause uterine rupture.

But hindsight is always 20/20.

After twelve hours, my uterus hadn't ruptured but my cervix hadn't ripened either. It remained rock hard and closed shut. I was still at two centimeters. My uppity vagina had iced the intravaginal pill and the cavalry led by Fabio, so they told me I had to take Pitocin.

I was defeated. By that point, I was pretty deep into the rabbit hole: It was midnight and I was at the hospital, with my name bracelet, wearing my backless gown. I could hear Mick Jagger talking me into it over the soothing sounds of my birth playlist, mainly dominated by the wordless giant, Mozart. So I took the damn Pitocin.

And. Nothing. Happened.

Nothing happened for six hours.

At six o' clock the next morning, my doctor came in before his morning run or tennis match (he was wearing workout clothes) and decided to take matters into his own hands, literally. He broke my water with something that looked like a chopstick. I felt labor pains instantly.

People ask: "What do contractions feel like?" Here's the best I can do: It feels like someone's gripping, tugging, and punching at your lower abdomen. With every tug, tsunami waves of electric shock spread through your body, crippling you with every set. I'm talking twenty waves per set, each one twenty feet tall, during a *Point Break*–type swell. Except there's not enough time to get back on your board before the next wave rolls in.

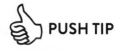

PUSH TIP

Booking an Induction?

If you're getting induced, book your appointment for first thing in the a.m. You will want to sleep in your own bed the night before. You could also save the fee for a night's stay.

If you're not into the surfing/*Point Break* references, here's a different one: "I felt like I was the lemon being crushed over one of those juicers," described Holly in "18 Women on What Contractions Really Feel Like" on nymag.com.

I endured feeling like a degutted citrus, still hoping I could get through labor without any more drugs. I decided that I would give it one hour. I stared at the wall clock for sixty minutes without any encouraging signs of progression. As soon as that little hand hit seven, I'd had enough.

Through contractions, you can't move, you can't speak, you can't even scream: "PLEASE GIVE ME THE FUCKING EPIDURAL!" So I whispered it instead.

If I go through this again, I need to remember that the anesthesiologist is not a genie who comes out as soon as you rub the magic lamp. That slippery fellow took another hour to get to my room. A lot of contractions happened during that time.

And by the way, I was surprised to find out that the epidural refers only to the shot on your spine, not the analgesic itself. But I digress.

While I waited to be sedated, I thought of my two BFFs who had pushed through labor without drugs—two times each! I wanted to be a badass like them. I felt like I had failed my own birth plan. Why do they call it a birth "plan" anyway? It's impossible to follow through every single step and even more impossible to not feel disappointed with yourself. I felt ashamed that I couldn't hack it. But I couldn't imagine pushing a baby through that pain. I'm in awe of everyone who does.

I'm the One Pushing... Right?

After the formidable epidural did its job, I was thrilled to breathe and smile through my anesthetized contractions. I was too relieved to feel guilty about it. I took solace in the birth MO of one of my other BFFs: "I've been a fan of drugs my entire life—why stop now?" I embraced the calmness that the epidural brought to me. I could've done a happy tap dance had my legs not gone to shit.

Besides numbing limbs, the side effects linked to regional anesthesia administered through an epidural are longer labor, increased risk of Cesarean section, and decreased chances of "spontaneous vaginal delivery."

Of course, when you're up on that bed, none of it seems "spontaneous." I suppose that means without the use of a vacuum or forceps rather than like a bout of barely-made-it-to-the-bathroom diarrhea. Wouldn't it be nice to spontaneously shit out your baby like that?

I was in a daze thinking ridiculous thoughts. From the waist down, my limbs felt like rubber. I hated this feeling almost as much as I had hated the pain. But the numbness was a small price to pay. My baby's dimmed heart rate was the high price. Just because I wasn't feeling the contractions didn't mean my daughter wasn't feeling them in utero.

Fun Fact About the Epidural

Dr. Leonard J. Corning, a neurologist in New York, was the first physician to use an epidural. In 1885 he injected cocaine into the back of a patient suffering from spinal weakness and seminal incontinence.

During contractions, the uterus is "flexing." It tightens, then it relaxes. Over and over again. This is supposedly more manageable during spontaneous contractions, as your body spaces the contractions enough seconds apart to gather a bit of strength between waves of gut-wrenching pain. But Pitocin-induced contractions can come so close together that sometimes babies can't recover quickly enough before the next squeeze.

Birth activist Doris Haire describes the effects of synthetic oxytocin (Pitocin) on the baby as "holding an infant under the surface of the water, allowing the infant to come to the surface to gasp for air but not to breathe."

During my contractions, my baby's heart rate slowed significantly. We tried to soothe my daughter by positioning me in all fours. It didn't work.

Our nurse had warned us that if something scary were to happen, a bunch of people would come into the room. What she didn't expand upon was how many fresh-faced, hip, millennial interns would get to witness the depths of my vagina.

But I didn't care. I was scared. My baby's heartbeat wasn't picking up. So they injected me with yet another drug, terbutaline, to slow down the contractions that had been prodded by the Pitocin, the gateway drug after all. This new medicine made me feel as if I had snorted cocaine letters spelling *"stop feeding me narcotics."* I felt like a cracked-out whore: I had taken four different drugs and was lying pantless in a spread-eagle position, being probed by strangers.

Thankfully, my husband's calm confidence was contagious, and in spite of the drug domino effect, I wholeheartedly trusted my doctor, nurse, and the hospital staff. I had to. Our lives were in their hands. In a short time and thanks to the high-octane dope, our daughter's heartbeat normalized.

At that point "the force" came over me. I was fully dilated and ready to push. But I couldn't do it after the drug snack pack and with my jelly legs. I told them to stop the drip on the epidural and anything else that was pumping through my veins. My doctor agreed.

I was calling the shots, I reminded myself. This was MY labor. I was the one pushing. And at last, it was time.

The doctor, still in his running shorts and sneakers, put a latex-covered finger on my perineum and told me to "push from the butt." So I pushed and pushed with my butt.

The doc and the nurse told me I was close. I thought they were BS-ing me. I had taken shits longer than this. Speaking of which, I don't know whether or not I shat during labor. My husband, faithfully by my side the entire time, can neither confirm nor deny this—he dared not look down. I don't blame him. I didn't want to look either when the nurse offered me a mirror. Some things are better left unseen. My husband did admit that his peripheral vision betrayed him a few times. I didn't ask further. Some other things are better left unsaid.

Finally, those twenty-five minutes of pushing came to fruition. I could feel our baby's head crowning out of my vagina. Let me put this in a way people with penises can understand: Pushing a baby out of a vagina is like pushing Barbie Skipper through the penile urethra. Wait 'til you get to the shoulders. Drugs or not, it hurts like a motherfucker.

Pushed, Unsealed, Delivered...I'm Yours!

After twelve hours of being at the hospital, five of them in active labor, our Sweet P and her placenta finished their journey out of my unsealed vagina and into the world. Thanks to my nurse, I got to hold her right away. The nurse had constructed a "landing pad" where she could clean the gunk (officially called vernix) off my daughter quickly before handing her right over to me. I also got to breastfeed her immediately, as planned, which I took as a gift. She latched onto my boob with the ease of a newborn puppy. She loved that thing so much, she didn't suck on anything else for first year of her life.

We did have to cut the umbilical cord right away because it was too short. I had wanted to keep her connected a little longer, but I got beat. A few times.

But who cared about the stupid birth plan at that point? I realized that my healthy daughter was the only part of my birth plan that truly mattered. Holding my daughter in my arms was worth every second of discomfort and agony I have *ever* experienced. I thought of the Rolling Stones' song again—the part about not getting what you want, but what you need. And my baby was everything I ever needed *and* wanted.

Those precious minutes rank higher in my life than a lazy hammock nap under a palm tree with a warm, salty breeze after a long swim. I felt at peace. I had no regrets.

Well, one.

I wish I had filmed this moment. Not the pushing carnage, but the beautiful outcome lying on my chest, bumping her head up and down like a baby turtle coming up for air. Her little hands with paper-thin nails and her red-marbled legs thrashing about as if she was ready for her first swim. The warm sunlight breaking through the window, enveloping my little family in a cozy shade of blue.

I don't want this one to ever fade from my memory, but already the corners of the picture are starting to blur. I need to stop thinking about it or I'll cry. I'm not a cynic when it comes to affection.

I was the proud mother of a healthy 8-lb., 6-oz., 23 ¼-inch baby girl. She was here. She was ours. At least for the next eighteen years.

And at last, the carnage was over.

Or not.

The Final Insult

Our family was in the room meeting our daughter when the nurse suddenly kicked everyone out. She had been routinely keeping tabs on my beat-up vagina and wasn't comfortable with the unusually large stream of blood gushing out of it. Something was wrong.

The nurse suspected I had a blood clot in my uterus and requested the midwife to come back into my room. *Dear Mary, Mother of God,* I asked to the heavens, *did you get a blood clot, too?*

Our midwife—who looked like a cat lady and not the fun, quirky kind with red rhinestone eyeglasses—slid on her rubber gloves. Without giving me any anesthesia, she went in there like I was the Operation board game, buzzing every second as she fisted my vagina—which, I may add, already felt like it had been plowed by a John Deere tractor.

Luckily, the epidural needle was still in, so I asked that they pump me with more drugs to get me through this Operation game. (I had come full circle in my war against birth drugs.) While digging around in my uterus, the lady somehow managed to reopen my Level 2 vaginal tear, so I had to get re-stitched.

I cringe every time I think of that woman. She was abrupt and careless. The entire time her hand was inside me, I focused on that baby sleeping in the see-through box across the room, wrapped in a white, pink, and blue blanket, wearing a ridiculous hospital-issued hat with a bow on it.

The thought of holding her again is what got me through.

Confessions of a Happy Mom

After it was all water under the vagina, I asked Abigail (whose advice I sought in *Chapter 8: Labor a la Carta*) to look into my medical transcripts. "According to your records," she told me, "when you presented to the hospital, you were already mostly effaced, two centimeters dilated, and at a negative-one station—certainly not an indicator that 'nothing was happening.' Rather, your baby was low enough to be putting pressure on your cervix and moving down. Dilation is not a reliable predictor of when a mom will start labor, but OBs still use it that way. My point is that had you not been dilated at all—hard posterior cervix, no effacement—that would have been a different story. I wish you had been given more options as to how to proceed post-date."

Chronology of My Induced Labor

From Pitocin to birth, my labor took less than twelve hours. And the contractions (a.k.a. worst physical pain known to womankind) didn't start until my water was broken by my bare-legged doctor. From that moment forward, it was 5 hours, 51 minutes, and 2 seconds to a Level 2 tear and "spontaneous" delivery at 41 weeks, 1 day. I only pushed for 25 minutes. The pushing part was the easiest.

10:00 p.m.	Admission.
12:00 a.m.	Cytotec pill.
4:00 a.m.	Pitocin drip starts.
6:00 a.m.	My water is broken with a chopstick.
7:00 a.m.	"I think I need the epidural, please."
7:15 a.m.	"Where is the epidural?"
7:30 a.m.	"Give me the fucking epidural."
7:45 a.m.	Finally got it! "When does this kick in?"
8:00 a.m.	*I'm drugged as hell. Fuck. Now I can't feel my legs.*
8:30 a.m.	Baby's heartbeat goes down. "We've got to give you something else to STOP the contractions."
10:00 a.m.	"You're fully dilated. Let's get you off drugs. I'll be back in a bit to deliver."
11:25 a.m.	"Let's get ready."
11:26 a.m.	"Push. From your butt."
11:51 a.m.	Baby is born.
1:04 p.m.	*"Oh Shit. You've got a blood clot. Let's call in the cat lady for a game of Operation!"*

SAT-Worthy Labor Vocabulary

When I started hearing all the labor terms, I might as well been trying to interpret Mandarin. And the numbers associated with them? They're worse than trying to remember geometry basics. I've tried to pare the info down as much as possible in hopes that you'll actually remember it and be better versed than I was when I gave birth to my baby.

Effacement

As labor nears, your cervix, previously long and thick, shortens and thins out with contractions. It basically "disappears"—or more accurately, becomes part of the uterine wall.

Medical staff measures effacement in percentages. When your cervix reaches 100 percent, that means it's ready for Baby to journey down it into the depths of the outside world.

Dilation

Besides being long and thick, your cervix starts out closed shut like a clam, to keep bacteria away from your baby. When the mouth is closed, dilation is at zero. When it's time to deliver, the cervix dilates up to ten centimeters to allow Baby safe passage.

Station

Think of train stops. Your baby has to travel down seven stations in order to exit, and each "station" is a measure in centimeters of how far down your baby has come into your pelvis. This is by far the most complicated number because it involves the use of negatives; also it's not entirely accurate, since the assignment is estimated, not measured.

The station starts at -3 (head is high and floating above pelvis), and as Baby nears the pelvis, it reaches -1. When Baby has made a temporary home in your pelvis, level with the ischial spines (bony ridges in the tightest part of your pelvis), he's living at zero station and is "engaged." This is also called "lightening."

> As Baby begins his descent to his final destination, he enters the positive station, escalating from one to three. Three means that Baby is at the gate (or crowning), ready for pick-up.

Looking back, I of course wish I would have labored without any drugs as I'd originally planned. Pitocin is sometimes medically necessary, but for us it was a choice and maybe I could've held out a little longer. As I saw it, I had three options: wait, induce, or schedule a C-section to cut to the chase (pun intended).

I went with my doctor's induction recommendation, mainly because I was afraid of the complications that could stem from having a post-mature baby. My baby did shit six hours after she was born, so who knows? Maybe if she had still been in utero, she would've breathed it in, gotten MAS, and spent her first hours in the NICU instead of on my boob. As a result, maybe she wouldn't have latched as well as she did and I wouldn't have nursed her for twenty-one months.

In retrospect, at the time of my daughter's birth, I was ill-informed. Maybe skipping the birth class wasn't the right decision. It was only afterwards (when I became obsessed with finding out whether or not what happened had been "kosher") that I learned what I should've known prior to birth-giving. I hadn't even been aware that I could seek out an acupuncturist to help me progress into labor; I wasn't clued in that Cytotec had any adverse effects; and I had never heard of terbutaline—which I've since learned is associated with serious side effects to Baby and Mom (though mainly after prolonged exposure).

Conversely, induction of labor (IOL) post-term *does* lower the risk of perinatal morbidity and infant mortality (the death of an infant immediately before or after birth). My doctor didn't bring this statistic up, probably because he didn't want to freak me out. And he did a phenomenal job of keeping me calm and delivering my baby. And for that, I will put my second baby (if there is one) into his capable hands.

Still. *What if, what if, what if...* I try to not let myself obsess over any of it. In the end, I did not feel cheated out of the labor experience because things didn't go as planned.

Despite the cat lady's brusqueness, I felt everyone in that room had my back and, most importantly, my baby's back. This was paramount. And in this case, it was true that "all's well that ends well." My baby was perfect.

My vagina was a different story. Someone in my "Breastfeeding and Returning to Work" course said that after delivering, her labia looked like hot dog buns. I wasn't brave enough to look at mine, but they felt like a smashed, overripe fruit. All my girl was missing was a cloud of flies hovering over her remains.

It took a while, but I'm happy to report that both she and my daughter are now walking and talking.

BRINGING UP BABY

Who Invited the Peanut Gallery?

W E LEFT THE HOSPITAL a day early. We had plenty of reasons to run out of there. I was bleeding through my pads like a harpooned whale and was being forced to urinate in a plastic mini-tub so someone could inspect my crimson fluids. As if splitting my vagina and being fisted in front of a crowd hadn't been humiliating enough.

We were zombies, wanting to bite to death all the people who came in and out of our room at all hours. One of our nurses tiptoed into our room in the middle of the night, woke up our baby, undressed her, and put her on a scale. I was outraged and unafraid to say so. The nurse patronizingly admonished me for being oversensitive.

We finally fell asleep again after she left, but not for long. An alarm made us bolt upright from our subzero-thread-count sleeping arrangements. The ear-bleeding beeps were

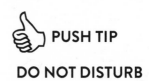 **PUSH TIP**

DO NOT DISTURB

If you choose to birth at the hospital, post a **DO NOT DISTURB** sign on your door through the night and tell your head nurse that if everything is going well, you'd like to sleep undisturbed.

coming from my IV monitor; I had run out of juice. Our baby was right next to it, and we were sure she had suffered permanent eardrum damage.

We'd had enough.

My OB/GYN signed off on the early exit plan even though our pediatrician and (good) nurse urged us to stay one more day. When we respectfully stuck to our guns, the nurse looked me in the eyes and warned me very forebodingly not to have sex for six weeks—that I could get pregnant again even though I was breastfeeding. I almost blood-peed in my giant pad. Who the fuck's thinking about sex after having a baby. It's not a question; that's why I ended the sentence with a period.

The nurse continued on with her advisories, trying to cram in as many instructions as possible as we were leaving. She was almost on her knees, begging me not to go. A veteran mother of four, she thought we didn't know what the hell we were doing. We dismissed her well-intentioned concerns and reassured her that we would be fine. How hard could it be, right?

And like that, our little family of three was released into the wild. My husband and I marched onward, thinking: *We've got this.*

We stupid, cocky motherfuckers.

The screenplay for this next scene would read...

```
CUT TO:

INT. CAR - PARKING GARAGE - DAY

New parents try to decode a strange device.
It's a car seat. They look like two big
dinosaurs with little hands trying to
detonate a sticky bomb.
```

The simple task of putting our baby in her car seat made us question our decision to leave the hospital early. Our T. rex hands pitter-pattered about, trying to prevent our child's decapitation by seat belt. We were taken by surprise at the emotional difficulty of moving our daughter's delicate limbs to fit inside this contraption. When our friends had a similar experience taking their baby girl home from the hospital, the dad even suggested—very gravely— that they give up and the mom hold the baby on her lap for the short ride. (Thankfully, they didn't end up partaking in that "joy" ride.)

Once our own daughter was secured in her car seat, I couldn't allow this sweet baby girl who'd crawled out of my vagina to sit in the back all alone, so I let Daddy chauffeur us across town while she clutched my index finger. I stared at her miniature hand, inspecting her soggy nails that were still soft (and smelly) from being pickled in amniotic fluid. Poor thing. She'd gotten my short, big-knuckled fingers with flying saucer nails. The same hands I got from my mom. It was a bittersweet discovery, because while her third-generation stubbies will never be seen in an engagement ring ad, they'll always remind me of the caring hands that raised me.

Mother (-in-Law) Knows Best

Back at home, our daughter slept most of the day, as my husband and I high-fived each other, repeatedly singing *"We've got this"* to the tune of MC Hammer's "U Can't Touch This." Oh yeah.

We breezed through the day 'til dinnertime. I was starving, and my Puerto Rican ass was in dire need of some spice after all that bland hospital mush. We ordered Chinese and I laid on the sriracha hot-chili sauce.

```
INT. IVETTE'S DINING ROOM - NIGHT

The Inquisition Panel, a.k.a. PARENTS-IN-LAW,
sit across from Ivette. They are horrified at
her cavalier use of sriracha. Finally, they
dare question her dietary choice.
```

```
                    MOM-IN-LAW
              (eyebrows raised)
         Are you sure you want to eat
         that?

                      IVETTE
                 (defensive)
         My milk's not in yet.

    In-laws exchange looks, but wisely keep
    eating their pale, mild Chinese food.
```

My in-laws left after dinner and soon came "happy hour." I wish this meant that my husband and I clinked cocktails and head-tilted to *"We've Got This"* while our newborn slept. For those of you who don't know what baby happy hour is yet, enjoy your peace while it lasts. This is the hour when your child goes berserk and there's very little you can do about it but shove a breast or a bottle down her throat 'til she passes the fuck out. It's like sundowning for infants.

Now, I'd seen some pretty scary sundowning firsthand when my Mamá María was in the hospital after her hysterectomy. But her crazy ass didn't hold a candle to her great-granddaughter.

In this particular instance, shoving my nipple down her throat wasn't making it better. So, because I was (am?) a stupid, cocky motherfucker, I told my husband: "She must be allergic to my colostrum!" (Colostrum is the gooey stuff, rich in antibodies, that your boobs leak out before the milk comes.) I kept trying to nurse my baby and she would latch on and then recoil in inconsolable tears, arching her back away from me. My heart was breaking in a million pieces and I didn't know how to glue it back together. I could tell that her little tummy hurt and I was desperate to make her feel better. I felt incapable and scared.

Why the fuck did we leave the hospital early?
We ain't got this.
At all.

We spent the second night as a family of three in bouts of hysterics interspersed with spells of sleepless exhaustion fueled by adrenaline and caffeine. (Experts agree that consuming 200–300 milligrams of caffeine a day is safe while breastfeeding. I found every single milligram to be completely necessary.)

I held it together that night (literally) until I plié-d down with my baby in my arms (did I say stupid?) and a rush of warm fluids exited my weakened vagina dam. I couldn't see anything in the dark, but I thought my stitches had ripped and that I was hemorrhaging to death. I was ready to dial 911.

Instead, I woke my husband and handed him our screaming daughter. "I need you to take care of her while I take care of myself," I told him.

He accepted her bravely in solidarity, but I'm sure he was thinking: *Don't be long; I still don't know how to change a diaper.*

I sat on the toilet, expecting to see Moby Dick emerge from my vagina. I was surprised to discover that I had only pissed myself. This is what happens to a pelvic floor during delivery. I squirted my wound with cucumber-infused witch hazel water and put on another hospital-issued lady-diaper. Some women think they are comfy. Me, I'm a tampon girl. Walking around with that body pillow wedged between my legs made me feel like I was going to the Barney Ball.

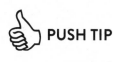 **PUSH TIP**

Pad Pops!

After delivery, douse your pads with witch hazel and stick them in the freezer. The cooling effect is almost orgasmic.

The next morning when we took our baby to the pediatrician, the doctor made me manually express my mammary gland. Loss of modesty aside, we learned that our baby had lost an entire pound overnight and that my milk had come in early on day two, full force and full of sriracha. I owed an explanation to the inquisition panel.

I felt so guilty. But I also hoped this didn't set any kind of precedent. I really, really hate to be on the wrong side of any argument.

It Takes a Village,
and There's Always an Idiot (Me)

If you don't get along with your mate's parents, I have terrible news: You're screwed. Now that you have given them a grandchild, they'll expect to be *very* involved.

Lucky for me, I didn't get beat in the in-law department. They're truly fantastic. In spite of some differing sociopolitical views, I have found surrogate parents in them and, having spawned from two divorced generations, a great example of what a good marriage can be. Just don't bring up gender-confirmation surgery and everyone gets along like Care Bears in the Forest of Feelings.

They're also excellent grandparents. They help out, and I don't mean just holding the baby when she isn't throwing a fit. They feed all of us. They clean. They redo the yard. They rock their crying grandkids. Often. Lovingly. The summer of our baby's birth, they moved across the country to be near us.

Now here's the much-awaited rub: My in-laws came with Teddy and Vinny, a pair of cute little fuzz-puff Pomeranians that I wanted to squeeze into furry balls and throw back to the Georgia backwoods they hailed from. Normally I love these dogs, but having a newborn in my home was nerve-wracking enough. These yapping little rascals provided a moving obstacle course every time I wanted to cross the house with my baby in arms. I detested their presence, and I held my poor in-laws responsible for making me endure the guilt that came with such meanness.

On top of the pesky Poms, my mother, two sisters, one of their boyfriends, my dad, and his wife (who doesn't like to be called Stepmom [I blame Cinderella for ruining the term] but has been in my life in a great big way since I was twelve) were also visiting to meet the first granddaughter on either side of the family.

Word to the wise, ladies: Do not have everyone come visit at the same time—*especially* if you have divorced parents.

We had a full house, and from a casting perspective, quite the fodder for a reality show under our roof. As they do in movie credits, I'll continue in order of appearance.

My father is a short, stocky-and-cocky Cuban man whose demeanor hints at Asperger's. He is extremely particular about air not hitting his neck and is often caught mumbling numbers into space or swinging an imaginary golf club. On the flip side, he's focused and quite good at everything he does. An engineer by trade, my dad can fix anything and is quite diligent. (Thank the universe, because my husband is not; it takes him six months to hang a picture in our bedroom.) While my dad was in town, he bought and installed a chandelier for our dining room and black-out blinds for the nursery. To hang the chandelier, he climbed up on our dining table and then sweated and cursed at the ceiling while we watched television. When focused on difficult physical labor, my dad is a cross between Donald Duck and a profane, disgruntled Popeye without the tattoos. He fought that chandelier until it was properly installed.

My dad also loves the token sitcom "pop in." He is generally oblivious to any sort of social etiquette, such as calling to ask if it's okay to stop by. I will never forget the first time it happened.

INT. IVETTE'S BEDROOM - EARLY MORNING

Ivette's husband enters. His face is as white as Casper's but not as friendly.

HUSBAND
Your dad is at the door.

I mean, let's not forget that my family is 100 percent Hispanic. Invading personal space is not a concept we understand; "overstepping boundaries" isn't in our vocabulary. I've had a conversation with every single member of my family while one of us was sitting on the toilet. Recently.

Yet there's a big upside to the cultural "familiarity." My dad and his wife were a huge help during their streak of unannounced visits. His wife prepared home-cooked meals for us and stocked our fridge. She even folded our clothes, which equally mortified and gratified me. I don't like people sifting through my underwear, but I appreciate when people help out without being asked.

Why?

I hate asking for help. I'm well aware that this is a problem. I'd rather complain about someone not helping than ask them to lend a hand. I also dislike being asked questions. Nothing sets me off like a string of inquiries.

Which is part of the reason my mom drove me absolutely bonkers. She'd ask how she could help, and then ask if she was doing it right, and did she need to do it again, and did she need to do it differently—because all I had to do was ask, you know? *Argh!* I loved being able to share my first days of motherhood with her, but she wanted to help so much that she sometimes got in the way.

It's a tragicomedy—no one can set you off like your own mother. Now that I have a daughter of my own, I'll get to be on the other end of the relationship. I'm sure my mom will get a kick out of that.

My two sisters were considerate and helpful around the house, and it was a treat to have them with me. But—and of course, there's a but!—they were intimidated by newborns. They were afraid to hold their niece. In fact, one of them didn't even stay long enough to build up the courage. The other one held her only while seated and under requested supervision. So I couldn't really dump my daughter into their arms and go take a bath.

Believe it or not, I would've killed for some time to take care of chores, too. Some books advise that family should help with housework and leave you to bond with baby. But for me, there was only so much bonding I could do—I confess it got a little boring. I was suffering from domestic blue balls.

Little did I know that this was the beginning of a very long journey of constant interruptions, unfinished projects, and learning to "let go" of my need for completing tasks and being organized. Every time I'd start alphabetizing my cooking spices, I was pulled away by my hungry daughter or by a relative requesting my assistance in helping me.

I wanted someone to hold my baby while I played in the kitchen. And if I couldn't have that, I wanted my daughter to myself. I was a little sensitive about sharing my baby. But I would also get upset if nobody wanted to hold her. Everyone was driving me nuts. I started looking forward to nursing breaks so I could get away from them all. But staring at the wall alone made me feel left out. I am well aware that I was acting like a world-class brat—and maniac. Blame it on the hormones, but it was really hard for me to be satisfied during the first three months.

I realized I couldn't hide away every time people drove me crazy, so I resolved to set boundaries. No open door policy in this house. Mi casa es *mi* casa. I took pains to carefully schedule visits or at least get my dad's wife to text me a head's up. I tried to never have more than two or three people over at the same time, and I politely suggested an end time *("We all need to nap when she goes down!"* I'd sing). Which of course required timing visits an hour or two before naptime. Most of the time, we didn't need to nap, but I wanted my house and husband to myself while our daughter was asleep.

I had to get my husband on board with the rules and regulations, so he would have my back when we needed to enforce the boundaries. I especially needed him to help manage his mother's obsession with our daughter. She hovers over our little girl, which is beyond amazing when I'm not around. But when I'm with my daughter, I get the helicopter coverage by association. My mom-in-law becomes Pepé Le Pew to my Penelope Pussycat. If I put my daughter in a stroller to take her for a walk, my MIL slides next to me, sneakers and ball cap on, ready to stroll along. I rely on my husband to kindly remind his parents that even though we love them so much and love how great they are with our daughter, we sometimes need our own time alone with her.

In fairness, I also serve as a buffer between my husband and my own drop-in family, who never seem to know when they've eaten all of our food and/or overextended their welcome. My mom would've moved in if we'd let her. And by all means, we're never having all three sides of the family (divorced mom/remarried dad, etc.) in town at the same time again. Ever.

Thankfully, besides their little annoyances—loving us too much (how dare they?!) and Grandmas' iPad addictions—our family allows us to be the parents we want to be. Which is ultimately all we can ask of them. (A quick aside, iPads should come with a warning label: *Following grandchildren while photographing with this device may result in new mothers injuring your hardware. In this event, no refunds will be issued.*)

The truth is that everyone we love drives us mad from time to time. And when you have a baby, they can feel like hemorrhoids in your butt. Even with those who are allegedly on board with your parenting philosophy, it's hard not to feel judged when they have strong opinions about everything. Breastfeeding, maternity leave, nap schedules, sleep training, baby-led weaning, religion, sexual preferences...the list will grow with the child.

Having family in town was rough. But you know what was rougher? When they all left. We were left to fend for ourselves.

Don't Sleep When She Sleeps

"The woods are lovely, dark, and deep.
But I have promises to keep, and miles to go before I sleep."
—*Robert Frost*

Those first few months were harder than I had expected. I loved my daughter infinitely, but sometimes she felt like a ball and chain. There's only so much you can do when you have to hold, feed, bounce, and change a baby 24/7. I was stir-crazy, like a bug inside a jar.

While my body was occupied with caring for her in a series of mind-numbing activities, my brain had the luxury (or torture) of being able to think about all the things I wanted to do but couldn't. Even mundane shit, like the lack of time to clip my toenails, would send me into despair. I couldn't seem to get anything done except during her early-morning nap, which was when I started writing this book.

Writing was the saving grace of my maternity leave and perhaps why I remained in relatively good spirits those first few months. It was hard not to just go back to sleep at daybreak, but this was time I carved out to do something for me. This is why I want to punch people in the face when they say "sleep when she sleeps." If I had done that, my home would be in shambles, my body wouldn't have bounced back as fast, and this book would never have been written.

Rest when you need to (and can) rest—not when she sleeps. Babies nap a lot, and naps are brief windows of freedom for a new mom. A freedom that will shut close before you get to fully enjoy the view.

If You Can Afford It, Pay for It

When you don't have family nearby, paying for services is not a luxury but a necessity. For us, hiring help has become a very well-worth-it financial outpouring. We have a team of sitters on speed dial, nicknames for our delivery guys, and a cleaning lady who comes in once a month. (Side note: She just inherited a quarter million dollars and is now richer than us. #onlyinla) Your body, your mind, your relationships, and your home deserve time. You can't do it all alone. And unfortunately, help ain't free. But I'd rather pay to get my house cleaned than buy a new outfit. Sanity, cleanliness, health, and the illusion of a life outside of "Mom" are my top priorities.

Like most families, we struggle financially, but I firmly believe that hiring a hand can keep darkness at bay. Having help with the house reduces stress and silly arguments over chores—both of which tend to double after a baby, just as your time and money decrease. It may seem like a splurge to get a sitter, but fifteen dollars an hour to go out on a date is way cheaper than paying a therapist. And if you're there, going to a therapist is way cheaper than a divorce lawyer.

Hell, I've been tempted to rent a call girl to service my husband. I keep telling myself, *Today I'll give him a BJ.* But it's like the pathetic diet procrastination curse: *I'll start on Monday.*

A Love Triangle

It's hard to quantify and verbalize what happens to a romantic relationship after a baby. Before I pushed our baby, I was worried that this little person would take away love and attention from me. I would no longer be my guy's girl, but one of his girls. But after she was born, this fear completely dissipated. We are a threesome and I feel right at home in the corner of this love triangle.

This is not to say that my relationship with my husband hasn't changed. In some ways it's stronger and in other ways...different.

I have to admit I miss fancy dinners and drunken karaoke in K-town. I long for the desire to cook us an amazing dinner and the energy to put out afterwards. I yearn for post-crazy-sex lazy weekend mornings filled with yet *more* adult-only cuddles. I'm sure he does, too.

Since baby, date nights and sexual encounters are like red carpet events we wish to attend but have been left off the guest list to. And when we do get the opportunity to partake in such occasions, we struggle to find energy, a sitter, and what to wear or not to wear. We still find time to "connect," but outings are a bit more costly and time-consuming.

About once a month, we'll treat ourselves to dinner and a movie. We'll map out the cheapest and closest theater/restaurant combo in order to minimize the expense. On most Fridays—our pre-baby built-in rain or shine date night—we sometimes have a nice dinner at home after we've put our daughter to sleep. Then we move to the couch, where we spend the next forty minutes deliberating what movie to watch. This decision-making process often ends with "I'm now too tired to sit through a movie," so we end up settling for a couple of *Seinfelds,* or recently *Brooklyn Nine-Nine*. (This is unlike Wednesday nights, which are thankfully no-brainers: *Law & Order: SVU* and *Chicago PD.*) Quite the fairy tale, don't you think?

Having a baby is a real test to romance. You're running on little sleep and frayed nerves while bearing hard-to-manage responsibilities and emotions. I've always had mood swings, but since getting back my period, it's like my body is going through global warming. I can be a raging bitch (is there any other kind?) or I can act cold and detached. I don't want to be spoken to, let alone listen to my husband go on one of his Larry David–esque rants. (That was a reference to *Curb Your Enthusiasm*—yeah, we watch a *lot* of TV.)

My husband gets easily annoyed at everything and everyone, including me. But it's a two-way street, baby. As previously mentioned, progressive inquiries drive me absolutely bonkers. Try to figure shit out before you ask me.

The other day I left my husband with our daughter so I could cohost a baby shower for one of my BFFs. Before I could get to the location, my husband had called and texted:

HUSBAND

Where's the diaper bag?

IVETTE

By the heater.*

*What I really wanted to say: "Where it always is."

1 MINUTE LATER

HUSBAND

Found it. Where's the sunblock?

```
                    IVETTE
            In the diaper bag.*

   *What I really wanted to say: "Where it
   fucking always is."
```

It's so hard to be nice to your partner when (justifiably or not) you really don't feel like it. Especially, when they are shaking your marbles!

As already established, I drive him nuts, too. His grievance list is pretty solid. I always lose my phone. Always. (True. I don't know how many phones I would've had to purchase if the "Where's My iPhone" feature didn't exist.) I constantly burn myself. (At least once a week, not even joking.) I stomp like an elephant around the house. (True.) I leave the kitchen faucet on hot and it has scalded him many times. (Unfortunately.) I'm never on his side. (Not true. Sometimes I am!) I'm super-defensive. (*I can't believe you just said I was disgusting!* He had only pointed out that I had toothpaste on my mouth.) I like to be the martyr. (I only regret that I can't clone myself to do more around the house.) I may be a tad passive-aggressive. (See previous example.)

We most certainly piss each other off. We yell at each other— a few times in front of our daughter. When I'm in the heat of it, I forget I swore to never do the bad shit my parents did when I was growing up. I push, push, PUSH 'til I get a reaction that maybe I'm not ready to deal with, and then I instantly regret it but don't know how to diffuse or apologize. I say cruel things I can't ever take back. And those are just the big fights. Most relationships are filled with little tug-of-wars that can threaten anyone's sanity.

In a perfect world, I wouldn't need to ask: "Can you take care of her while I shower?" Instead, I'd like to hear: "You must be exhausted and I'd love to spend some time with our daughter, so I made you a bath. And don't worry about dinner; I've got it covered. And, yes, sweet cheeks, I'll do the dishes, too." If that were to happen, I'd be like: "Don't wake me up, because I'm Kate-Fucking-Middleton right now!" Though to be fair, I'm sure Prince William delegates all those courtesies to their servants.

But to us middle-class commoners with children, our households are a constant intense course in negotiation tactics. By the time our kids hit college, we should be able to successfully procure hostages from the world's most hostile, inflexible captors.

Keep fighting the good fight, fairly. Negotiation can help strengthen a parenting team. The end game is to reach an agreement between both parties in which nobody feels shortchanged. This is important because when someone does most of the baby "heavy lifting," the scale tips too far and someone starts to feel resentment. But it's a tricky thing because if I ask for something to get done, I may get accused of nagging. But if I don't say anything, he'll never know what I need from him.

I have to constantly remind myself that, much to my chagrin, my husband can't read my mind. Sometimes I have to tell him *exactly* how he can help me get through the week. I feel awkward and condescending, but at least I'm helping us avoid Ivette-the-Nag yelling at him for not thinking to offer to pick up food on the way home after a particularly trying day. I can blame my partner for not addressing my needs, but I can't fault him for not guessing them.

I learned this the hard way. I was building up so much resentment because I felt like I did everything on top of caring for our baby. And my husband would be the first to admit that I did *do* most things. I planned, managed, cleaned, inventoried, nursed, hunted, gathered, and cooked. Plus, I worked! *I'm bringing home the bacon, too,* I thought. *So why do I also have to cook it?!*

I was working myself ragged and I felt a little like the default parent. Every morning it was just me caring for our daughter. In my husband's defense, he didn't wake up early because he had the "afternoon shift": He took care of our daughter every afternoon from 4:30 to 6:30 p.m. until I came home from work. In my defense, I had to care for her every morning from 4:30 a.m. 'til 9:30 a.m. before heading to the office. One-two-three-four...FIVE hours! I would've loved for him to get up and help me get ready for work in the morning. I would've killed to just have an "afternoon shift." Instead, I was working and nursing full-time (more on that juggling act later). Not to mention, I would get home from work and my husband would thrust the baby into my arms as soon as I walked through the door and hide behind his laptop to catch up on work for the next hour while I nursed. Would it have killed him to keep me company? Or talk about my day? Or get dinner started while I fed our baby? But he had to work—that's the plight of a freelancer with a home office. Now, I can relate. But then, me, the martyr, suffered silently.

On the weekends, to give my husband some me-time, poor old me would haul our daughter everywhere instead of asking him: "Can you watch her while I go work out?" Or even responding to him: "Yes, I really *do* want you to come with us to the farmers' market" when he offered. Instead, I would say: "No, we're fine," because I knew he didn't really want to go. But by sparing him an afternoon outing, I was doing harm to our relationship because I was harboring resentment against him.

One day, I finally said (or yelled, rather): "Sometimes I feel like a single parent!" That was hurtful and it wasn't true. I instantly wanted to take it back. He is a very involved father; we're equal partners when it comes to parenting. But he had no idea I felt shortchanged. He was honestly doing the best he could, and he thought I was doing just fine because that's what I had led him to believe!

Once I communicated to my husband exactly what I needed him to do for me—for us—he did it. Sometimes begrudgingly, but he did it. We started to take turns in the mornings. He became more involved in errand-running and dishwashing, and he tried to effect a more positive attitude towards his loss of freedom. Becoming a dad has taken a lot of my husband's time and it's really hard for him to be okay with this. And it's baby steps for me, too, because I'm coping with my own loss. Instead of screaming it to the four winds like he did, I swept it under the rug and tried to forget what it felt like to not bear the cross of parenthood.

The few times I allowed myself to dwell on it, I felt guilty about missing my fly-by-the-seat-of-my-pants life. After all, I had really pushed (pun and all) to be a mom. So why would I all of a sudden feel tied down by the responsibility and the mundane routine of it all?

I'm learning to be more honest about how I feel and speak up when something bothers me instead of bottling it up and taking it because I think that's what wives and mothers are supposed to do. That's not healthy, or fair, or even a good example for our daughter. Not to mention it's very backwards of me.

I feel compelled to advocate for a shift in our preconceived notions of what a parent is supposed to be in this modern world. I mean, why is it that when someone brings home the bacon, the other is expected to cook it, when in actuality they've been working just as hard and probably longer, running the household? Also, how come only a "homemaker" gets to "make" a home? These are all questions that may be worth discussing with your partner before your family grows. (More on convoluted domestic terminology in *Chapter 14: The Baby, the Boss, the Home, & Your Lover: Juggling Life While Exclusively Breastfeeding.*)

Speaking of bacon, it's important to get on the same page when it comes to money. How much to save, how much to spend, where, and how often.

Another biggie amongst new parents is that after years in a relationship, they realize that their parenting styles are completely different. Someone is invariably stricter, less religious, more scheduled, less organized, or healthier than the other. These issues can grow and really hurt a family.

I'm way more anti-junk food than my husband will ever be. So if he's eating M&Ms and wants to give some to our daughter, I really try to look the other way. I think they're terrible, but are they worth the fight? They don't even melt in her hands! Plus, he's her daddy and he's got a say in what she eats, too (even if it has [gasp!] Yellow #5 and high-fructose corn syrup). Gotta pick my battles.

When it comes to really serious matters like religious views or school choices, it's a good idea to schedule a talk in a neutral location and remain open-minded. In the end, you both want the same thing: the best for your child.

"What's Love Got to Do With It?"

Everything, actually.

In spite of our new parental hardships, my husband and I have somehow managed to remain in love. It's a struggle, but we consciously rebel against the adage "This is just what happens when you have a kid." We try not to give up on our appearances just because we got hitched. We try not to forget romance just because we made a baby. We make a point of spending quality time with each other, even if it means dining at a cheap BYOB pizza place so we can afford a sitter that night. And when we sit across from each other, we try to talk about something other than our child. This is *so* hard, especially when you run out of things to say but have a phoneful of cute pictures to "Aww" over. But she *can't* be the only thing we have in common.

Besides our daughter, the biggest thing my husband and I share is our sense of humor. I don't think we would've fallen in love and stayed in love without it. We laugh with each other and at each other all the time. I don't know how anyone survives life without laughing at it.

It's difficult to manage disappointments in life—professional, personal, and domestic. As far as our careers and family matters, it is great that we can be there for each other "for better or worse." But when it comes to our domestic life, well, we really just try to work on our expectations. My husband doesn't assume that I'll cook, wash, or clean (I impose all of this on myself). But he at least pretends to be impressed when he comes home to a tidy house. He's very appreciative of everything I do. Every night, he makes a point of tucking me into bed. He also thinks I haven't aged since we met in 2001, so he gets bonus points for being blind as a bat.

We also took away a couple of important lessons from our requisite Catholic pre-marriage class. One, to never start an argument with the pronoun "you." "Rather than accusing," the veteran marriage volunteer told us, "say how your loved one is making you feel." Instead of saying "You're not listening to me," say: "I feel as if I'm not being heard." It's a very small adjustment in communication technique, but it makes a big difference. Another tactic that's probably in every Marriage for Airheads booklet but is still easy to forget: Try not to bring up old arguments or missteps, especially during fights currently underway.

The key word in all of this is "try." Sometimes we fail miserably, but we don't give up. We get back up, ready for another round. We're not here to fight each other. We're here to fight for our Hollywood ending.

TO VACCINATE OR NOT TO VACCINATE?

Is There a Question?

INITIALLY, I WASN'T SURE WHAT I WOULD DO. Having read some of the anti-vaccine propaganda, I was pretty hesitant to commit to a vaccine schedule. Yet, I wanted to make an educated decision for my daughter. So I took a tempestuous trip into the well-documented sea of vaccines.

Anti-Vaccine Arguments

Anti-vaccine movements claim that vaccines can cause brain damage, are responsible for infant mortality rates, and cause autism.

The anti-vaccine movement got traction in 1998 with a fancy article published in *The Lancet,* a U.K. medical journal, way before Jenny McCarthy rallied the troops. The article was co-authored by Andrew Wakefield, who was at the time being paid by lawyers to be an expert on an alleged vaccine injury case. His article linked the MMR (Measles, Mumps, and Rubella) vaccine with causing autism and bowel disease.

In 2004, ten out of the twelve study's co-authors issued a retraction, citing insufficient data. But Dr. Wakefield stood strong in defense of his study. The same year, *The Sunday Times* (London) cited *The Lancet* editor Richard Horton as saying: "[*The Lancet*] should not have published the study...Wakefield's links to litigation against the manufacturers of the MMR vaccine were a 'fatal conflict of interest'" (Brian Dreer, *The Sunday Times*, Feb 24, 2004). In 2010, *The Lancet* officially retracted Wakefield's article.

After twelve years of subsequent research, no one could find a link between autism and the MMR vaccine. Dr. Wakefield still defends his report entitled "Ileal-lymphoid-nodular hyperplasia, non-specific colitis, and pervasive developmental disorder in children" and has a bit of a cult following amongst the "anti-vaxxers." However, he has yet to replicate his findings.

The "vaccine causes autism" argument still gets tossed around even though studies continue to indicate that there is no correlation between vaccines and autism. In May 2014, Autism Speaks reported that a meta-analysis involving 1,266,327 children reaffirmed that vaccines don't cause autism. "If anything," cited the article, "immunization was associated with decreased risk that children would develop autism, a possibility that's strongest with the measles-mumps-rubella vaccine."

I read and read, but I simply couldn't find sound medical evidence that correlated vaccines with autism or mortality rates in infants. The most alarming side effect cited was brain damage; however, it is so rare that there's no hard proof that the vaccine was actually to blame.

Perhaps the biggest anti-vax argument is that some studies that prove vaccines' safety do not take into account the effect of toxins, such as aluminum and formaldehyde, being injected intramuscularly versus being injected intravenously or ingested. The reasoning here is that a toxin injected into a muscle has a higher chance of absorption and a lesser chance of excretion, which arguably also helps the vaccine to be effective. However, there are no conclusive scientific findings on this aspect of vaccination, either.

There are a few risks worth noting, however, which is standard with every medical intervention.

Vaccine Side Effects

Vaccinating our children is scary. We're shooting them up with a germ concoction through a needle. Vaccine side effects include serious allergic reactions or seizures—enough to give parents pause and cause to consider not vaccinating. A serious allergic reaction may include wheezing, hives, dizziness, heart palpitations, and deafness; in most extreme cases, certain vaccines have been linked to permanent brain damage. These extreme allergic reactions are very rare and vary from vaccine to vaccine.

The CDC estimates that the risk of a serious allergic reaction from any vaccine is one in one million doses—the same odds as dying in a bathtub. To put it in further perspective, according to the National Safety Council's Odds of Dying chart, one is statistically over five times more likely to be struck by lightning and fifteen times more likely to die from a hornet, wasp, or bee sting.

The most serious confirmed side effect of the rotavirus vaccine is intussusceptions: a bowel obstruction that may require surgery but is most often treated with an X-ray procedure in children. This occurs once in every 20,000 to 100,000 infants vaccinated. You have better odds of dying in air-and-space transport. Minor side effects can include fatigue, headache, nausea, fever, soreness, and a mild rash.

Besides all that, it's simply heartbreaking to hold your child's little body and stare into her scared eyes while she gets pricked with a needle. I dread shots as much as any parent.

It's important to pay close attention immediately following vaccination, because an allergic reaction usually happens within a few hours after the shot. Be ready to go to the hospital at the slightest indication that something isn't right.

Although it's scary, the advantages to be gained with a single shot benefit not just our children, but our communities.

Herd Immunity

Perhaps the most important factor to bear in mind is that the only way to keep our community free of deadly diseases is to keep our herd immunity in check.

I think we often forget how bad outbreaks were in the not-so-distant past. We take for granted that we live in a well-developed country where—thanks to vaccines—most serious diseases have been eradicated. Yet, our herd immunity has been compromised by the vaccine-phobia permeating our modern society.

WTF is herd immunity?

I do hate being called a "herd," but this basically means that a group of us bipedal animals living in the same area have been made immune to a specific contagious disease. However, when a significant amount of the population lacks immunization, the herd immunity threshold can dip to unsafe levels and make us all more susceptible to a contagious disease.

"The epidemiological concept is based on this logic: If the chance of an infectious person crossing paths with a susceptible person is very low—as would be the case in a population whose vaccination rate is at or near herd immunity—then even a very infectious disease may not be able to spread within their population. The more infectious a disease is, the greater the immune proportion of a population must be in order for herd immunity to protect susceptible population members" (*WBUR's Common Health,* August 2013).

Even though I advocate for everyone living their lives through their own experiences, this is one issue that does affect others, and our babies are amongst the most susceptible since they're not immunized. Here is a sobering statistic: From 2000 through 2014, 277 deaths from whooping cough were reported in the United States. Almost all of the deaths (241 of the 277) were of babies younger than three months of age, who were too young to be vaccinated and were relying on herd immunity to keep them safe.

Vaccinating your child can save other parents from suffering the most painful, unimaginable loss: that of their child.

Stats Speak Louder Than Words

Here is a little bit of history on vaccines, their ingredients, and the diseases they've helped eradicate:

VACCINE EFFICACY

Smallpox

The smallpox virus was responsible for an estimated 300 to 500 million deaths during the twentieth century—over three times more casualties than WWI and WWII combined. We lost two million people to smallpox in the year 1967 alone.

It took us almost two hundred years to fully endorse a smallpox vaccine after its creation in 1796 and eradicate this "red plague" that is believed to have originated in 10,000 B.C. Google Image Search smallpox and tell me you're not happy someone made a vaccine to get rid of that shit.

Whooping Cough

Before the DTaP (diptheria, tetanus, and pertussis) shot was routinely given to infants, about 9,000 people in the United States died each year from pertussis (whooping cough). After the vaccine was introduced in the 1940s, the number of reported cases gradually fell from roughly 200,000 to 1,010 by the 1970s. But over the last few decades, cases of pertussis have risen. In 2012, 48,277 instances of whooping cough were recorded. And as mentioned previously, from 2000 through 2014, this disease was to blame for 277 deaths in the United States.

Measles

Worldwide, about 20 million people get measles each year and 146,000 of them die from it. Measles is so contagious that 90 percent of unvaccinated people will catch the virus if they're exposed to it. Without the vaccine, it is estimated that 4 million cases of measles would occur in the United States every year. Thanks to the MMR vaccine, we kept the number of cases down to 50 for a long time. However, in 2011, 222 measles cases were reported—the highest level in fifteen years. Then, 2014 saw 23 measles outbreaks in the U.S., including one large outbreak of 383 cases. In 2015, the Washington State Department of Health confirmed one death due to measles. There hadn't been one since 2003. Most recently, in July of 2016, there were over 22 cases of measles reported in Arizona.

Polio

In 1952, during the worst recorded polio epidemic in the United States, 3,145 people (including 1,873 children) died and 21,269 suffered mild to disabling paralysis.

Rotavirus

In the United States, before the rotavirus vaccine, this virus caused about 2.7 million cases of severe gastroenteritis in children, leading to almost 60,000 hospitalizations and around 37 deaths each year.

DISPUTED INGREDIENTS

Thimerosal

The flu vaccine is the only vaccine that currently contains thimerosal. Thimerosal is a mercury-loaded preservative that breaks down into ethylmercury. However, ethylmercury doesn't accumulate in the body like methylmercury, the toxin found in some fish that can be harmful when consumed in large amounts. So eating fish is more dangerous, is what I'm saying.

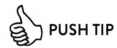 **PUSH TIP**

Thimerosal

Single doses of the flu vaccine are available without thimerosal. If you'd like to do without it, ask your doctor if it's available to you.

Aluminum

Aluminum adjuvants (substances added to a vaccine to boost the body's immune response to it and enhance its efficacy) do have the potential to be harmful, but aluminum salts, aluminum phosphate, and aluminum potassium sulfate have been properly tested for safety and have been used in vaccines for over seventy years. The following vaccines contain aluminum: Hep A, Hep B, and DTaP.

The amount of aluminum gels or salts in vaccines is less than what children get through breast milk or formula. However, the body absorbs more aluminum when injected in your muscles than when ingested, so this is still a valid cause for concern. I do hope we can develop a safer adjuvant than this for our vaccines.

Formaldehyde

Formaldehyde is used in vaccines to inactivate viruses and bacterial toxins being injected. Once the bacteria or viruses are killed, the formaldehyde is diluted, leaving small traces of it behind. The following vaccines contain formaldehyde: DTaP, Hep A, Hep B, Hib, meningococcal, IPV-IPOL (polio), typhoid (except the oral version), and some influenza shots.

It is well known that inhaling formaldehyde in copious amounts can be fatal and that long-term exposure to it may result in respiratory illnesses and/or cancer. This is why we fear it. However, this gas is a natural by-product of decomposition and even has antimicrobial and antifungal properties. Our body typically produces more formaldehyde than the amount found in vaccines and is able to metabolize and eliminate this substance fairly quickly.

Antifreeze

There is no antifreeze in vaccines. Yeah, some people do think that.

SAFETY TESTING

Vaccines must undergo ten to fifteen years of testing before they can get approved. Then, the vaccine goes through the FDA to ensure its effectiveness and safety. Then the CDC, AAP, and American Academy of Family Physicians decide if it can be released.

Challenging the Middle Ground

Some people believe in vaccines but think that the recommended schedule is too aggressive. In 2007, Dr. Robert Sears of the famed Sears family of doctors published *The Vaccine Book: Making the Right Decision for Your Child*, which encouraged parents to stretch the vaccine schedule into twenty-one visits instead of thirteen. Maybe he was trying to inspire parents to get their children vaccinated eventually (better late than never), but his alternative vaccination schedule "which he has admitted he simply made up— has been discredited by pediatricians, researchers, and a growing body of medical research" (Tara Culp-Ressler, thinkprogress.org, February 2015).

There is no proof that side effect risks are minimized by postponing vaccines. In fact, the University of Washington recently conducted a study that revealed that measles-containing vaccines are twice as likely to cause a febrile seizure when given late. Furthermore, delaying vaccines can make babies more vulnerable to contracting easily preventable diseases. Call me crazy, but I trust the federal government's recommended vaccine schedule and the team of experts who put it together.

That said, vaccines like the HepB shot—which is usually administered at the hospital soon after your baby is born—could be safe to postpone if the birthing mother doesn't have hepatitis B. Hepatitis B can cause a lifelong infection, serious liver damage, and even death; however, this disease can only be contracted from sharing drug needles, contaminated blood transfusion, sexual activity with an infected partner, or from an infected mother during childbirth. Heeding our pediatrician's advice, we opted out of the HepB shot at the hospital and delayed it 'til our daughter was three months old. If you wish to do the same, make sure you convey this to the hospital staff as they can be HepB vaccine syringe–friendly.

Many parents also opt out of the chicken pox and flu vaccines. These diseases aren't that dire; in fact, most of us have survived them. Also, the flu shot is only 50 to 60 percent effective. Keep in mind, however, that although rare, a really bad flu could kill you. Also, before the vaccine was available, varicella or chicken pox killed 100 to 150 children a year and was the leading cause of necrotizing fasciitis, a flesh-eating bacterial infection. Varicella could also be very dangerous for pregnant women who haven't been immunized. Their babies could be born with "congenital varicella syndrome." This may cause scarring of the fetus's skin and problems with arms, legs, brain, and eyes.

BIG NO-NO!

Pregnant women should not get the chicken pox vaccine as it could cause serious fetal complications. Yet another reason to keep our herd immunity in the safety zone.

The Bottom Line

Whether or not you agree with our current vaccination mandate, it is a fact that vaccines do save lives.

I recently visited a mother whose unvaccinated son died of measles when he was seven. As we looked at his last school photo, a young boy with straight dark hair and a big white smile standing in front of a bookcase, my heart broke for his mother whose own heart will never mend.

Mari, one of my BFFs who pushed two babies without drugs, spent a terrifying week at the NICU after her firstborn got infected with pertussis. Her daughter pulled through, but I know how scary that was for them. Actually, I *don't* know. Only they do. Do you really need to be put in that situation to become a believer?

Parents often argue: "This is my child; I'm doing no harm to others." But unless you live in a bubble, your decision *does* affect others. By not vaccinating your child, you're lowering the herd immunity. Think of it as an invisible cloak that protects all of us. The truth is that even though vaccines have successfully combated terrible diseases, they're not 100 percent effective for everyone, and not all of us can be vaccinated due to factors such as autoimmunity issues. But if 95 percent of us are vaccinated, we can protect those who aren't.

Say that in twenty years they discover a vaccine against AIDs... would you want your grandchildren to take it? And that's not even a great parallel, since AIDs is not an airborne or even water-borne disease, so it's therefore harder to contract than, say, smallpox.

Another consideration is that we don't know what congenital diseases could stem off unvaccinated children when they become adults and have children.

"There's a bigger picture in this vaccine debate," explained my cousin, a pediatrician with a specialty in epidemiology. She's way above my pay grade on this subject and has a medical clearance that comes with ten-plus years of studies in the field. She blew my mind when she told me that it may be possible for congenital diseases such as rubella to pass on to fetuses and cause fetal death, blindness, or deafness. Of course, this hypothesis is still being researched and tested, but the point is that the medical community is concerned. We won't know the full repercussions of not vaccinating our kids until they have children of their own.

Can vaccines be improved? Absolutely. But as I pored over the research, I became a believer. To me, the benefits outweigh the risks. I'd rather take all the tears from the injection, the aluminum, and the slim chance of an allergy than see my daughter battle a fatal disease like the measles, polio, whooping cough, or any other virtually "contained" disease.

I have a bit of a conspiracy theorist in me like the best of us, but I don't really think pharmaceutical companies and the government are cohorts in an Enron-like scheme. In fact, most of the federal funding for vaccines goes to universities for research, not to the pharmaceutical companies that *do* profit from vaccines. It is a business, but no one is tricking us into spending money to avoid whooping cough.

If your child does suffer from a vaccine allergy or a severe side effect or can't be vaccinated for other medical reasons, we owe it to you to keep our herd immunity levels in the safe zone. We all want the same thing: healthy children.

So, how do we keep them safe?

We all have our own children to care for and our own roads to pave. I do hope that 95 percent of us agree on immunization so we can keep a lid on outbreaks for the other 5 percent.

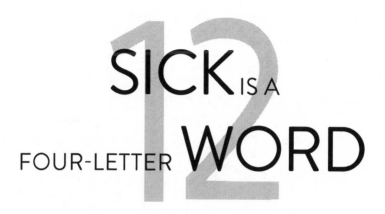

SICK IS A FOUR-LETTER WORD

Fussing Over a Fussy Baby

IT WAS A PUKE-FEST. My five-month-old daughter was the protagonist victim in this dramatic affair. The doctor suggested giving her Pedialyte, but she wasn't drinking out of a bottle or allowing me to "syringe it." As a workaround, I was told to wait thirty minutes after each vomit to put her on my boob and then to pry her away after a few short gulps. It seemed cruel, but since she wasn't keeping anything down, I couldn't allow her to drink to her heart's content. It was a rough Friday night.

Then it got rougher.

My daughter's nanny/aspiring writer Dear John–ed us via email at two in the morning (which we read during a puking/nursing break), to inform us that she'd just happened to land a job as a showrunner's assistant on a Netflix series and had stopped by during the night to drop off the car seat and house keys in the garage. We needed to find somebody new by Monday.

When your baby gets sick, it pours.

Taking care of a sick baby can make you feel helpless. It's hard to see your sweet daughter struggle with a cold, a broken arm, or even teething, and not be able to make it go away. Add in sleepless nights for all involved, and helplessness gives way to another Dante-worthy circle of hell.

During these trying times, try to remember that this, too, shall pass.

I've compiled a list of seven ailments that are common in babies, with some basic info on how to handle them. **This general guide is not intended to replace medical advice given to you by an actual doctor.**

The Unlucky Seven

#1 *Gastroesophageal Reflux (GER)*

I imagine GER to feel like the soured-whiskey burning taste I get when I burp after eating something super greasy (read: Puerto Rican frituras). GER is very common in newborns because the muscle flap between the stomach and the esophagus is still "a baby" and has yet to learn to properly keep acid down in the stomach. GER often causes babies to spit up and/or vomit. Overall, it causes a general malaise that makes your baby prone to fussiness. Hopefully, your baby's GER (and fussiness) is temporary and not an indication of Gastroesophageal Reflux Disease (GERD), which is a long-term condition.

Should I call the doc?

Absolutely. Especially if your baby's GER is affecting her sleep or weight gain, or she seems to be in a lot of pain. Medication and/or probiotics may be necessary. Plus, you'll want to rule out the possibility of GERD.

How can I make it better?

Feeding your baby lesser amounts with greater frequency may reduce GER, because if the stomach is not full to the brim, so to speak, food is less likely to rise back up to the esophagus. During feeding, prop your child diagonally so that fluids travel down with gravity; also make sure that Baby is not gulping a lot of air and that you burp her often and correctly (behind the belly). After feeding, place your baby on an incline or upright position; baby carriers and stationary swings are particularly helpful with this.

If you're feeding your baby formula, try a different kind to see if he responds better to the new brand. If you're nursing, keep tabs on what you're eating. It's possible your baby is sensitive to all that chocolate milk, as mine was.

Our baby wasn't diagnosed with GER or GERD, but when she demonstrated discomfort after feedings, I changed my diet to alleviate her symptoms. First, I went dairy-free for a month. After that, I introduced yogurt and then cheese but avoided milk entirely for a year. This did the trick for us. I know of other moms who had to give up soy, as well, during breastfeeding.

We also gave our daughter drops of gripe water. Gripe water is made out of fructose, ginger extract, fennel, baking soda, and chamomile. There isn't any solid evidence to support gripe water's efficacy, but it did seem to sporadically help—though we often wondered if it just had a placebo effect on us. She seemed to really like the sugary taste, and we were thrilled to have her swallow anything that wasn't from my boob. At one point, I even considered feeding her breast milk one milliliter at a time through a dropper, too, but that would've been ridiculous...*right?* (Eight ounces equates to two hundred thirty-six milliliters.) Anyway, we stopped using gripe water after reading that it could introduce bacteria, cause allergies, and irritate a baby's intestines, even though she never had an ill reaction to it.

My pediatrician recommended I dilute chamomile tea, but I never got around it. (More details coming up in *Homeopathic Schomeopathic...Abuelita en la Casa!*)

#2 *Fever*

Fevers are a sign that your baby's immune system is fighting bacteria or a virus. They can also be a reaction to a vaccine. A high temperature can make your baby tired, miserable, and fussy.

While most fevers run their course without medical intervention, the symptoms that accompany a fever need to be minded: Baby's discomfort, hydration level, and skin and eye color, and the duration/frequency of the fever.

Most pediatricians consider anything over 100.4°F to be a fever. Dr. Paul C. Reisser, author of *Focus on the Family Complete Guide to Baby & Child Care*, asserts that "temperatures as low as 96.8°F or as high as 100.4°F are not necessarily abnormal."

I often find it hard to figure out if my daughter has a fever because the accuracy of thermometers varies from butt to armpit, and amongst different thermometers. Because of this, if your baby has a "borderline" fever, it's tough to assess the exact temperature.

When in doubt, it's wise to err on the side of caution. I once took my daughter to the doctor just to have them take her temperature. She didn't have a fever, but I was happy to have the confirmation. Don't ever be afraid to be that parent.

Should I call the doc?

It is always advised that you reach out to your health care professional to run through the symptoms accompanying the fever.

Definitely seek medical attention if:

- Your baby is under six months and has a rectal thermometer reading of 100.4°F or higher.
- Your baby has a fever over 104°F, regardless of age.
- Your child's temperature persists longer than twenty-four hours if he's under two, and seventy-two hours if he's older.
- Your baby is lethargic, looks pallid, has a stiff neck, seems sensitive to light, or appears to be in extreme discomfort.

Taking the Temp on Thermometer Choices

Thermometers have evolved, but in my opinion, they still haven't created a perfect, easy-to-use device that doesn't upset your baby. It's usually a pain in the ass to get Baby's temperature in any form because babies don't like to be prodded. And who can blame them?

Here's the skinny on what's available:

Infrared Thermometers: These don't require contact with the baby in order to take a reading. These puppies, which cost up to $60, read the thermal radiation emitted by your baby and can even sync up with your phone. They are considered accurate; however, the jury is still out in the rectal-reading-favoring medical community.

Digital Thermometers: These require minimal contact to take baby's temperature via the ear (a tympanic reading) or forehead (temporal artery). We got a temporal one and I needed another master's degree just to use this gadget. They cost anywhere from $25 to $50. Some experts advise against ear thermometers, deeming them inaccurate.

Axillary (Armpit) and Rectal Thermometers: These require the most "prodding," but they're the most straightforward for an old-school analog mama like me (though they're all digital now). A rectal thermometer is supposed to be the most accurate, but the "shock value" is hard to overcome—even if the doctor says the "baster" is way thinner than a poop! It is not recommended to use a thermometer orally or axillary once it's been used rectally, so don't try to double-dip.

- Your baby's skin feels cold and he is drowsy and limp, but his face, hands, and feet are pink. (These signs could indicate hypothermia.)

- Your baby shows signs of dehydration: dry mouth, a sunken soft spot, not drinking fluids, and fewer wet diapers (i.e., not urinating frequently).

- Your child is not responding to a proper dose of fever-reducing medication.

- Your baby's fever drops and then spikes again.

- Your baby's fever is accompanied by an unexplained rash.

- Your baby has a febrile seizure—he becomes unconscious and twitches uncontrollably.

- Your baby has an immune system condition such as sickle-cell disease or cancer, or is taking steroids.

- Your baby still seems "off" in spite of the fever subsiding, and you just feel that something isn't right.

How can I make it better?

Infants have a hard time regulating their body temperatures, so they need all the help you can give. Besides administering an appropriate dose of infant fever reducer (if your doctor agrees), you could also bathe your baby in tepid water and make sure he's getting enough formula and/or breast milk. If your child is older than six months, you can give her a tablespoon of purified water **between** feedings. Do not exceed more than four tablespoons per twenty-four hours.

BIG NO-NO!

Water Intoxication

NEVER WATER DOWN BREAST MILK OR FORMULA, and never give water to a baby under six months old unless advised by a trusted physician. This can cause hyponatremia (water intoxication).

#3 *Ear Infection*

Ear infections are fairly common in babies because the tube connecting the nasal passages to the middle ear is short, making it easy for snot (and viruses or bacteria) to travel from nose to ear. Fluid then accumulates in the ear, breeding germs that press against the eardrum.

There are three types of ear infections: inner, middle, and outer. Each can be either viral or bacterial. Only bacterial infections are treatable with antibiotics.

Inner ear and middle ear infections are the most common and usually develop in conjunction with a cold.

An outer ear infection, or swimmer's ear, happens when water gets trapped inside the ear and breeds bacteria. It is usually treated with antibiotic eardrops. An outer ear infection may also be caused by fervent efforts to clean the ear, because abraded skin can become a foothold for bacteria. To safely clean your child's ears, gently wipe them with a dry cloth on the tip of your index finger.

It's hard to tell when your baby has an ear infection because babies like to tug at their ears. They may be tugging because they just discovered the extra appendages, or it could be due to teething. Telltale signs of an ear infection are fussiness, difficulty sleeping, a fever, and/or a stuffy nose. Also, your baby may get really upset when you try to lay him flat.

The best way to properly diagnose an ear infection is to visit the doctor. Alternatively, some moms learn what an ear infection looks like, invest in an otoscope, and diagnose their own children. But I leave that stuff to the professionals.

Should I call the doc?

Yes. An ear infection gone awry can lead to a ruptured eardrum—which, thankfully though, is usually less problematic than it sounds. Although rare, repeated ear infections may cause hearing loss, which could in turn lead to speech delays.

If the infection is bacterial, your doctor may prescribe antibiotics, but if it's mild, your doctor may suggest letting it clear out on its own.

How can I make it better?

You can ease the pain with an infant-appropriate pain reliever. Never apply a hot compress or insert anything into your baby's ear. If it's a viral infection, you can do anything you would to fight a common cold (see next).

As a preventative measure, at the onset of a cold or stuffy nose, I stuff a rolled-up towel under our daughter's mattress so that she's at an incline. In this position, fluids are less likely to fester in her head and throat, which can help avoid an ear infection or keep it from worsening.

#4 *Common Cold*

Colds happen. They usually stem from viral infections that inflame the respiratory system, including the nasal passages, which produce a lot of mucus. Symptoms can be treated to lessen the suffering, but the cold has to run its course. Antibiotics do not kill viruses; however, a cold may weaken the immune system, allowing a bacterial infection to grow, in which case antibiotics *are* needed.

Should I call the doc?

During the first three months, it's particularly important you *always* seek medical advice for a cold. Regardless of age, if you've waited it out but the cold won't go away or has worsened, or if your baby has lost weight, ring the doc. A cold may just be a cold, or it could indicate a bigger problem such as a respiratory illness or whooping cough.

Seek medical assistance immediately if your baby has difficulty breathing, blue lips, blue nails, a wheezing cough, a high or recurring fever, and/or thick yellow-greenish mucus. If your child suffers from an immune deficiency, call as soon as you see any symptoms at all.

Your pediatrician may prescribe nasal drops to help your baby breathe. They may be crucial to dispense before each feeding so that she can breathe through her nose while she eats through her mouth.

How can I make it better?

Once my baby made it to age one and I got my mama training wheels off, I became more confident in dealing with colds. My methods combine our doctor's advice, OTC (over-the-counter) medicine, breast milk, and some of my *Abuelita's* remedies.

BIG NO-NO!

OTC Cough and Cold Medication

NEVER GIVE COLD MEDICINE TO A CHILD UNDER AGE FOUR. An overdose could be fatal. The medicines and healthcare products regulatory agency (MHRA) advises to steer clear of OTC cough and cold medicines altogether until a child is six years old.

If our daughter seems to be in any kind of pain or has a fever, we give her infants' Motrin (since she's over six months old now). We also rub her chest with Vicks VapoRub. I know it could irritate her skin (it doesn't) and obstruct airways (that doesn't seem to happen either), but I love how the minty smell brings back memories of my own mom rubbing my chest with it. My daughter also loves the rub-a-dub-dub ritual. If you're nostalgic like me and choose to go this route, never put Vicks VapoRub under your baby's nostrils or anywhere else but on the chest. And wipe your hands afterwards—that shit stings if it gets in her eyes and you definitely don't want it in her mouth. An alternative to this is Vicks BabyRub or, better yet, an organic eucalyptus rub. You can even make your own using coconut oil with a few drops of eucalyptus and lemon essential oils.

When my daughter is sick, we run a humidifier with a bit of eucalyptus oil in it, and give her warm, steamy baths infused with patchouli and lemon essential oils. These oils can also help ease the body aches that accompany a fever. If (and only if) she's painfully clogged up, we suction and then squirt nasal spray in her nostrils; note that doing this too much can further irritate the nasal passages. Last but not least, if you're breastfeeding and fighting the same cold, you'll pass your antibodies on to her, so try to keep it up if your body allows.

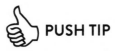 **PUSH TIP**

Washing your and Baby's hands often and thouroughly is the most effective way to keep colds at bay. Hand sanitizer is recommended to be used sparingly, only when soap and water are not available.

#5 *Influenza (Flu)*

This virus is extremely contagious, and I have taken my daughter to get flu shots since she was six months old. At age two and a half, she got influenza symptoms along with all the other kids under age three at her daycare. I really can't say whether or not the flu shot lessened the impact, but it obviously didn't prevent it.

The flu is a respiratory illness caused by any of the strains of the influenza viruses (A, B, or C). In babies, it usually presents itself with the loss of appetite and interest in play. Then comes a fever, which lasts from three to seven days, a stuffy or runny nose, a cough, and lots of crankiness. The symptoms overlap with those of a cold, so unless your baby's doctor performs a flu test, it's hard to know whether your baby has the flu or a cold.

Should I call the doc?

Yes, especially if your baby is a newborn, has an immune deficiency, has difficulty waking up and interacting, doesn't seem to be getting better after a couple of days, refuses to eat, and/or has a steady fever (see also fever recommendations above). The flu can develop into bronchitis, sinusitis, a middle ear infection, or if bacteria becomes involved, pneumonia. Watch out for any wheezing, difficulty breathing, and severe, persistent coughs.

How can I make it better?

To prevent the flu, you can get your kid a flu shot each year and wash his (and your) hands often, especially after hanging out in public playgrounds. Some essential oil blends also have antibacterial properties and may be used in the home to fight germs (more on essential oils to come). If he still gets the flu, you can do everything you would to alleviate a cold (above!).

#6 *Diarrhea*

Crap. Literally. Not only is your poor child shitting his guts out, but you have to wipe it. Or in some instances, wear it. (I've heard horror stories of being sprayed with confetti-string poop, and I'm quite thankful I've not been initiated in this way.)

This messy event is defined in the medical community as a condition in which stools become looser than normal and/or come out more often. Diarrhea is usually the result of a virus or bacteria in the intestinal tract; food intolerance; or an allergic reaction to food or medication. Diarrhea can last up to ten days and is sometimes accompanied by its sour compadre: vomit. And unfortunately, you can't plug both holes and hibernate 'til your baby gets well.

The major concerns with diarrhea are that it may cause dehydration and/or that it could be an indication of a more serious long-term problem, such as a food allergy or intolerance.

Should I call the doc?

Yes, especially if your baby is under a year old. And absolutely call if (a) the diarrhea comes with a high fever, abdominal pain, or vomiting, (b) the stools contain grease, mucus, or blood, or (c) your baby exhibits any signs of dehydration. Also let your doctor know if blisters, scabs, or redness spread around the anus or butt cheeks.

How can I make it better?

Don your hazmat suit, try to make your baby as comfortable as possible, and make sure he's drinking enough fluids. Don't forget to pay extra special care to your baby's butt. To minimize rashes, spray the area with water to clean off excess residue before wiping.

Be mindful of sanitation. Crap spreads a lot of diseases and you don't want anyone else to get sick. Wash both your and your baby's hands after every cleanup, and disinfect the changing area.

Double-check with your doctor, but in our experience, probiotics can help settle gut flora. We like the brand Culturelle Kids and it comes in powder form, which you can put in Baby's drink or food depending on his age.

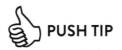 **PUSH TIP**

Pedia-Pops and More

Turn Pedialyte, breast milk, or formula into popsicles for your baby. This is particularly helpful during teething or if your child is having a hard time keeping food down.

Important: My friend who is a nurse adds: "Cold water and ice can cause dehydration, as the body needs to warm up the fluids for ingestion and absorption, so it's important to make sure she is also drinking room-temperature liquids."

#7 *Constipation*

While not as unsavory as diarrhea, constipation can cause a lot of discomfort all around. It's never fun for Baby to pass a hard poop—and for parents, to see Baby in pain or worry he isn't getting enough food because he's lost his appetite.

Newborns poop once a day on average, but irregular bowel movements are perfectly normal. Constipation is also fairly common after babies begin to eat solids (anywhere from four to twelve months). Your baby's system will usually regulate itself, but your doctor may prescribe treatment.

Should I call the doc?

Yes, if your baby is a newborn or shows symptoms of abdominal distention (protruded stomach), is vomiting, has a fever, and/or has blood in the stools. Also ring for help if your baby has been clogged up for more than three days, so your doctor can help determine if she is eating enough.

If you see blood, do call the doctor, but don't fret too much. Likely, a hard poop scratched the rectal wall. And if your doctor prescribes an enema (more in this "issue" below), those walls may repair themselves faster than it takes you to disinfect your shit-sprayed nursery walls.

How can I make it better?

In some cases and depending on your baby's age, your doctor will recommend laxatives, probiotics, and/or an enema—the latter of which will cause a hose of shit to fly out of your baby's butt and deck the walls (with rows of poddy, *fa la la la la*).

If your baby is breastfed, it's possible that Mom's dietary intake or a medication such as codeine could be affecting baby's bowel movements. If your baby recently started drinking milk or a new kind of formula, it may be wise to test other sorts or go back to her regular diet to see if the bowel situation improves.

If your baby is eating solids, you can try feeding her puréed prunes or adding a couple drops of flax seed oil to her oatmeal or drink. It's best to steer clear of bananas, rice cereal, and anything high in iron, which may contribute to the constipation.

Homeopathic Schomeopathic... Abuelita en la Casa!

My Mamá Gloria had an antidote for everything: rubbing on butter and salt to cure a "chichón" (goose egg); gargling warm water with salt to ease a sore throat; having a tablespoon of lemon and honey to fight a cough; applying camphor oil to clear up congestion; ingesting milk of magnesia to loosen up them bowels; sipping oregano tea with a sprinkle of salt or eating a lemon squeezed over banana slices to tighten them up; and my personal favorite: pouring cinnamon-and-vanilla infused steamed milk over sugar and raw egg yolk, and then mixing it up for a delicious elixir that always eased my menstrual cramps.

During teething, Mamá rubbed her daughters' gums with rum. Possibly mine, too. And although I'm not about to give my daughter her first taste of booze, I frequently use a lot of my *Abuelita's "remedios"* in my home.

Even with naturopathy and homeopathy (both alternative medicines but not to be confused, as the former is supported by science and the latter not so much), it is recommended to always consult your doctor prior to administering any holistic treatment to your child.

Honey & Lemon

A few drops of honey make the lemon go down! If your child is over age one, give her equal parts of lemon and honey in a tablespoon. Lemon dries

BIG NO-NO!

Honey is not recommended for children under age one, as it can lead to botulism, a rare but very serious disease.

up congestion and honey helps fight coughs. When choosing honey, seek dark, raw, and/or unrefined and be mindful of portions because, chemically speaking, it's the same thing as sugar (a.k.a. Frenemy #1).

Garlic

Garlic has antiviral, antifungal, and antibacterial properties. It's particularly great raw, which you can hide in a yummy homemade pesto for your toddler to gobble up in his pasta primavera.

Mullein Garlic Eardrops

Mullein is a plant whose flower is used to make medicine. The chemicals in mullein are believed to fight influenza, some viruses, and some bacteria. And since garlic is the shiznitz, manufacturers have bottled the two together and made the concoction available at most health food stores.

Mullein garlic eardrops are believed to help alleviate the symptoms of an inner or middle ear infection. However, this is not proven, since when applied in the ear, the liquid may not be able to reach the infection. **ALSO NOTE: These eardrops are not recommended for swimmer's ear and could worsen it.**

With our doctor's consent, we used these drops once on our daughter and it did seem to alleviate her ear infection. She hated them though and the garlic smell was quite robust, which also helped keep vampires at bay.

Chamomile Tea Drops

Lukewarm, diluted chamomile tea administered via drops *between feedings* may help tummy muscles relax and soothe your baby to sleep. Invest in a high-quality organic or reputable brand, and don't exceed two ounces (four tablespoons) in a twenty-four-hour period. You don't want your baby to get filled up on tea or put in danger of water intoxication. Stop using if you notice a rash. Definitely consult your doctor before trying this if your baby is under six months old.

Hair Dryer for Swimmer's Ear

Stand a foot away from the ear and air dry on *cool* setting. This may help evaporate water trapped inside the ear. I wouldn't use this on a baby, but I would try it with a toddler.

Cucumber for Mild Swelling

It's like a spa visit for Baby! You can put a fresh, cold cucumber anywhere you find minor swelling to help soothe Baby's skin. Stop immediately if a rash or irritation occurs.

Olive Oil or Coconut Oil

I used this on my baby's head when she had cradle cap (which is like newborn dander—not a big deal, just gross). Following doctor's orders, I rubbed in the oil, used a brush to loosen the flakes, and then shampooed. Voilà!

If you wanna drink up the benefits, cold-pressed and unrefined coconut oil has many valuable fatty acids, such as lauric acid, which have been shown to kill harmful pathogens (bacteria and viruses). I take a teaspoon of coconut oil in my coffee every morning.

Elderberry Syrup or Sambucus Nigra

We've recently adopted elderberry syrup as a cold-busting aid. Elderberry is believed to help boost the immune system and to reduce inflammation and viral symptoms, including the flu.

BIG NO-NO!

No studies have been performed to prove elderberry is safe for pregnant or breastfeeding women. Take special care to steer clear of it if either you or your baby has an autoimmune deficiency.

ESSENTIAL OILS: DYI HEALING BLENDS

by Claire Chandou Broussard,
Aromatherapy Student and Young Living Essential Oils Distributor,
Hollywood, CA, Mother of Two

Over two hundred references to aromatics, incense, and ointments are made in the Old and New Testaments of the Bible! How else do you think Noah got all those animals to fall asleep in his ark?

Essential oils (EO) have been used for thousands of years and in many cultures for the treatment and prevention of illnesses. The Egyptians were some of the first to use aromatic EO in wellness, beauty treatments, food preparation, and religious ceremonies.

Usage

Essential oils are pure extractions from flowers or plants, often used as alternatives to traditional cleaning, beauty, and medicinal products. Thanks to over-the-counter availability and a growing understanding of their benefits, essential oils are making a comeback.

Essential oils can be taken topically, aromatically, or even internally, depending on the type of plant source they are extracted from and the purity of the oil. Because they're highly concentrated extracts, a few drops go a long way. Three to five drops of EO to 140 ml of water or carrier oil is a pretty standard ratio for topical and aromatic use.

Thanks to electronic diffusers, aromatic oils are the most popular type. Diffusers cold-steam an oil-infused basin of water into the room, providing the health benefits of oils through inhalation. You can also place a couple drops of essential oil into the palms of your hands and inhale the essences directly. This is great for clearing a stuffy nose, relaxing for sleep, and alleviating sinus pressure.

If you're not into your entire home smelling like patchouli, applying essential oils topically may be a better option for you. You can add your preferred essential oil into a carrier or base oil such as coconut, jojoba, sweet almond, or olive oil to use as lotion or ointment. Some oils are safe to ingest; if so, this will be noted on the label with instructions. **Do not ingest otherwise.**

Brand

Choosing the right brand of oil can be overwhelming. It's important to seek high-grade therapeutic oils from a reputable company that sources their products directly from farms. Low-quality oils may be diluted, thus compromising their beneficial elements.

Blends

Hundreds of oils are available, but some of the more popular ones are lemon, lavender, and tea tree. These oils are commonly used topically during pregnancy and baby care to soothe, stimulate, and heal both Baby and Mom. I used EO in many different ways through both my pregnancies and with my babies. They are still staples in my home.

During pregnancy, parts of your body you never knew could hurt get sore—especially at night, when finding a comfortable sleeping position is nearly impossible. To soothe my body and help me rest, I rubbed copaiba-lemon-and-lavender-infused coconut oil on anything that felt achy. This homemade ointment serves as a pain reliever and muscle relaxer. It's also excellent for relaxation, massage, skin irritations, and overall contentment.

After giving birth, to recover from those long newborn nights, I diffused peppermint and lemon in my bedroom in the mornings as a natural awakener. I've heard some people apply it directly to the temples to stay alert while driving! **Please note that per the warning box on the next page, peppermint oil is not recommended for use during pregnancy or directly on babies;** however, there are many safe oils you can use to care for little ones!

The best thing about using essential oils during pregnancy and with babies is that they can be very effective in alleviating common cold symptoms or even fussiness.

Here are some of my go-to blends:

Eucalyptus + Lemon
These two oils are known to relieve nasal congestion—quite beneficial for a baby who can't blow his nose. Diffusing these two essential oils in a stuffed-up little one's room helps him catch some Z's. You can also add a few drops of lemon to coconut oil and rub on a sore throat.

Eucalyptus + Pine + Lavender
During the day and/or at the onset of congestion, I diffuse these oils or mix them with a carrier oil to apply to my children's feet.

Lavender + Wild Orange + Chamomile
To help my family fall sleep, I spray these oils diluted in purified water on our pillows, which reduces anxiety. Lavender alone helps with headaches and can even be mixed into honey or coconut oil to create an ointment to treat burns or scratches.

Citronella + Lavender + Tea Tree

These oils together make a great air purifier and laundry boost! I put a couple of drops of this blend into my kids' wash loads to get all those stinky smells out. This keeps my washing machine smelling fresh and eliminates that mildew smell that can easily build up. This practice was especially great during the baby stage when curdled milk and poop was on everything.

Chemistry 101

The cool thing about essential oils is that you get to be your own chemist: you can create countless combinations. Because while the oils themselves have specific historical and time-tested benefits, it's up to you to find the perfect combination that brings wellness to you and your baby.

BIG NO-NO!

The following essential oils should be avoided by pregnant women:

basil	clove	marjoram	rose
blue cypress	coriander	melissa	rosemary
camphor	dill	myrrh	sage
carrot seed	fennel	nutmeg	sassafras
chamomile	ginger	parsley	thyme red
cinnamon bark	jasmine	peppermint	wintergreen
clary sage	lemongrass	pennyroyal	wormwood

Also check for safety guidelines on the proper use on infants and young children.

Safety Precautions

When using essential oil on a baby, always dilute into a carrier oil such as olive oil. Before applying anything directly onto your skin or your child's, do a patch test on the underside of the forearm to ensure the oils won't cause an adverse reaction.

If an EO starts to burn your skin, DO NOT APPLY WATER. Water will only make it absorb quicker and deeper. Instead, use a carrier oil to flush and dilute it. **The exception is your eyes.** If, for example, you accidentally spill some on your hands and then rub your eye, you *can* rinse your eye with water. Or you can simply let your own tears flush it out. Either way, spoken from experience, it will sting like an inferno.

Over-the-Counter Pain & Fever Reducers

If your baby is older than three months and with your doctor's prior consent, you may judiciously determine whether or not to give him medicine for a fever or to alleviate teething pain. If you choose to medicate, use an age-appropriate pain reliever and follow dosage instructions according to your baby's weight. Never increase recommended dosage or mix medications without your doctor's guidance.

There are three types of OTC painkillers and fever reducers: aspirin, acetaminophen, and ibuprofen.

Aspirin

Most experts agree that aspirin isn't safe for children under eighteen, and everyone concurs that it is terribly unsafe for anyone under two years of age. So my advice: skip it!

BIG NO-NO!

Giving aspirin to children under two can cause a rare but serious disease called Reye's syndrome, which causes swelling in the liver and brain. Though it is FDA-approved to administer aspirin after age two, it is advised to withhold it from children under eighteen, especially if they're recovering from chicken pox or the flu.

Ibuprofen

If your baby is six months or older, you can administer ibuprofen. Ibuprofen has anti-inflammatory benefits, which is well-suited to easing pain from an ear infection. Do note that overuse of ibuprofen has been linked to gastrointestinal bleeding and kidney damage.

Acetaminophen

Acetaminophen has become synonymous with Tylenol, but it's used in a wide variety of drugs. Acetaminophen is the only safe fever reducer for babies six months or younger. Do note that acetaminophen has very few anti-inflammatory properties and that it is not recommended for children with asthma. It has also been linked with liver toxicity when used in inappropriate dosages.

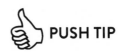 **PUSH TIP**

Opt for Fruity and Clear

I'm usually anti–fake sugary shit, but when it comes to medicine for my daughter I choose fruity and clear. I learned this the hard way.

Administering bad-tasting chalky pink medicine to my one-year-old proved to be messy and traumatic. I had to chase her, pin her down, and force-feed her with a syringe. Judging from the quantity of screams and pink-stained evidence at the crime scene, I doubt she ingested the prescribed dosage.

Selecting a clear, tasty medicine would've saved clothes, furniture, tears (mine and hers), and bruises (all mine!)

Anti-Antibiotics

Our daughter contracted an ear infection and a fever that lasted five days. It was hell. Because the prescribed antibiotic (amoxicillin) didn't seem to be reducing the infection and the fever persisted, our doctor had us switch to a stronger one (Augmentin—amoxicillin combined with clavulanate). But then, as the fever went away, an awful red rash broke out on her little body. The doctor diagnosed her with roseola, a mild viral infection common in kids under two.

The doc advised us to continue the Augmentin regardless to treat the ear infection—and because not finishing the course can lead to antibiotic resistance. But it pretty much destroyed our daughter's gut flora. Our poor daughter looked like a giant zit and had terrible diarrhea, to boot.

During this time, I had to travel with her from California to Puerto Rico—a twelve-hour, two-plane journey. Once the rash breaks, roseola isn't contagious anymore, but people surely thought I was smuggling disease in the form of a baby. I thought I was putting in purgatory time.

I learned three things from this experience: (1) It's very difficult to diagnose a baby, (2) Sex Ed & Prevention classes for teenagers should include air travel with sick children, and (3) antibiotics are a punch to the gut and a double-edged sword.

An antibiotic is wonderful when it's needed. However, antibiotics are sometimes prescribed unnecessarily and/or in inappropriate doses. They are also being injected into farm animals and passed on to their by-products that we consume (which is why I recommend buying antibiotic-free organic and/or grass-fed dairy, meat, and poultry in *Chapter 6: My Green Alter-Mama*). As a result, relentless bacteria have become resistant to antibiotics, putting common infections at risk of becoming untreatable. These antibiotic-resistant infections, MRSA (methicillin-resistant *Staphylococcus aureus*), are commonly referred to as superbugs, and they are a serious problem.

Professor Dame Sally Davies, chief medical officer for England, was quoted on *Medical News Today* saying: "In twenty years' time, we could be taken back to a nineteenth-century environment where everyday infections kill us as a result of routine operations" (September 2014). Women are particularly vulnerable to being infected at the hospital after giving birth or having a C-section.

"WHAT I WISH I WOULD'VE KNOWN ABOUT MRSA"

by Jessica Racioppo Freeman, Freelance Marketing Executive, Los Angeles, CA, Mother of One

When I departed our well-reputed hospital in Los Angeles five days after an emergency C-section, my baby was thriving and I was recovering about as well as anyone can after major abdominal surgery—with plenty of drugs. By some stroke of the gods-smiling-down-on-me luck, my newborn was nursing like a champ and even sleeping really well! Lucky me!

Almost exactly two weeks later, I couldn't wrap my head around why my recovery seemed to be going in a southward direction. It started with just plain fatigue—which frankly, seemed like a normal by-product of the sleep-deprivation coma I was in from frequent nighttime nursing sessions. All of the nursing books I had read had me so freaked out about getting mastitis (an inflammation of mammary gland tissue, usually due to a blocked milk duct) that when my extreme fatigue culminated in a 104 fever and chills that kept me under my down comforter over Memorial Day weekend, I was simply relieved because my boobs seemed fine—it couldn't be mastitis. So I assumed it was just the flu.

My husband, however, knew something was wrong and we were off to urgent care and then to the emergency room, where I spent a full day away from my daughter and husband (which is a big deal when you are nursing a newborn!) receiving intravenous antibiotics for what I soon learned was a superbug (MRSA) I had contracted during my daughter's birth. I had no idea that when the C-section performed is a *true* emergency, the doctors don't always have time to conduct the standard skin-sterilizing procedures before incision, so superbugs are a common side effect.

Months later, after seeing two infectious disease specialists, I was on the road to a slow recovery. It took almost a year for the disease to clear, and three years later, I am still dealing with ramifications from the hard-core antibiotics I took to kill it.

I can't help but think that if just one nurse at the hospital (or my OB) had warned me that contracting a bug like this was even a possibility, I would have been aware of the symptoms and could have headed down the road to recovery a lot sooner.

Due to this escalating issue, physicians are increasingly cautious about prescribing antibiotics. So don't be surprised if your child's pediatrician suggests waiting it out to see if an infection clears up on its own. When mine does, I generally abide by the recommendation. Our doctors went through a lot of schooling and testing in order to be able to legally prescribe or not prescribe medicines.

In Doc We Trust

I believe that the trained professionals I've selected as care providers have my kid's best interest at heart. And so, with their help and guidance, I get to choose what's best for my child.

However, this doesn't mean I trust them *blindly*. I know my daughter better than anyone and I always follow my instincts. In fact, my daughter was born with torticollis (a condition where the head persistently turns to one side). When we brought up the potential issue to our doctor at her three-month appointment, I saw a "these overzealous first-time parents" look in her skeptical eyes right before they rolled against her pastel-shadowed eyelids (we used to call her "clown face" based on her makeup preferences). Only after much insistence, did she finally concede to us and diagnose our daughter with torticollis.

Catching this condition right on time and starting the appropriate physical therapy avoided delays in our daughter's motor development.

We switched doctors shortly after that.

If a doctor makes you feel uncomfortable, or worse, dismisses issues that are important to you, it's time look for other professionals in your network. As parents, we need to question things that don't seem right to us and to always strive to find the best option when treating our children.

That said, I get concerned when our savvy parent culture acts like we always know better than doctors and teachers. So yeah, trust them, just be judicious about it.

Read On!

Eat, Sleep, Poop: A Common Sense Guide to Your Baby's First Year by Dr. Scott W. Cohen

A quick, informative read, written by a pediatrician and first-time dad. It's one of the few "medicine" books that didn't seem preachy, was mildly humorous, and was written in layman's terms.

The Baby Book: Everything You Need to Know About Your Baby From Birth to Age Two by William Sears, M.D., and Martha Sears, R.N., with Robert Sears, M.D., and James Sears, M.D.

A popular all-encompassing heavyweight, this tome includes info on breastfeeding, introducing solids, developmental milestones, and even babyproofing.

New Babycare by Miriam Stoppard

I really liked the layout of this book: super-organized and a breeze to flip through to find a specific topic. Easy to read for a non-scholar.

Your Baby's First Year by American Academy of Pediatrics

Pediatricians often recommend this APA-endorsed volume. It's a comprehensive practical guide to your baby's first year and a great investment for your reference library. In spite of its length (700+ pages), this book makes for a fast read.

Gentle Babies: Essential Oils and Natural Remedies for Pregnancy, Childbirth, Infants and Young Children by Debra Raybern

This is a great introduction to the magnificent world of essential oils for all the homeopathic-enthusiast parents out there.

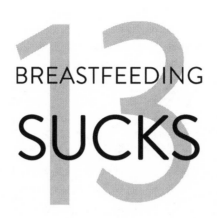

BREASTFEEDING
SUCKS

Pumping's Just Another Word for

Nothing Left to Lose

B REASTFEEDING HAS ALWAYS SUCKED. It is documented that back in the 1750s, about 90 percent of Parisian women hired wet nurses to feed their babies so that they could return to much-needed work. IIf pre-revolutionary women couldn't afford the time to breastfeed, how can we??

In the first year, I breastfed my daughter 49,769.7 minutes, equivalent to 829.5 hours or 34.6 days. After that, I stopped tracking the minutes on my phone app, but I kept nursing her until she was twenty-one months old (about 37,327 additional minutes—but who's counting?). That's a lot of time spent being milked.

As a mother of three breastfed babies, Hanna Rosin wrote in *The Atlantic Monthly:* "When people say that breastfeeding is 'free,' it's only free if a woman's time is worth nothing." If I had been paid minimum wage in the state of California, I would've made $7,465.46 for my first year of breastfeeding. Way more than formula would have cost.

Pro-Choice

As a sleep-deprived new mother with sore nipples, resentment, and guilt over that resentment, I embarked on a quest to understand the breastfeeding craze. I suspected it was one of those campaigns that had gotten out of control.

The breastfeeding movement initially grew fists to fight the aggressive and manipulative marketing of formula in the late '70s and early '80s. Like many honorable movements, it bred a few zealots.

I'm specifically talking about so-called "lactivists" who say that giving formula to your baby is comparable to child abuse. I find this to be offensive to adoptive parents, fathers of all kinds, and biological mothers who don't breastfeed. I get it: Formula isn't for everyone. But neither is breastfeeding.

The pressure to breastfeed is one of the biggest stressors some mothers face. We are often made to feel at fault if there's something wrong with our milk supply. We're bullied into ordering costly drugs across the border that rhyme with expensive champagne just to "get that milk going." We're pushed to keep nursing, even if our dry and butchered nipples are becoming fossilized. We're asked to push through mastitis, no matter the pain. Worst of all, we're downright shunned if we outright *choose* formula over this liquid gold that oozes from our breasts like lava from an erupting volcano. (I was surprised to find out that breast milk doesn't come out in one even stream; it bursts from your nipples like fireworks.)

Breastfeeding advocates are right to broadcast the many benefits of breast milk; however, I begrudge when they make parents feel inadequate or sinful for using formula. Let it be clear that I also object to nurses peddling formula to aspiring breastfeeders. I resent any attempt to steer us moms from our goals, and any judgment for the paths we pursue.

Dispensing "mommy guilt" is not a modern issue. Women have been giving each other shit since the dawn of time. In 1792, Mary Wollstonecraft, known as a woman's "advocate" of her time, publicly shunned the non-breastfeeding mama in her article "Vindication of the Rights of Woman." She stated that a non-breastfeeder "scarcely deserves the name of a wife, and has no right to that of a citizen." She paralleled breastfeeding with educating children, because obviously we all learned our ABCs with a hooter in our mouths. Even back then, the scarlet letter was hung on those ladies who, for whatever reason, did not breastfeed their children.

Some two hundred years later, marketing made formula hip and lack of education turned it into something dangerous. At that point, breastfeeding crusaders came to the rescue to enlighten the masses. But a few may have stacked up their soapboxes too high. Some went as far as to cold-shoulder women who struggled to continue breastfeeding after returning to work. My mom-in-law, a nurse who breastfed in the times of formula, had to manually express her milk into bottles to keep her baby fed while she worked long shifts at the hospital. She called the Leche League, hoping to hear: "Hang in there—it'll get easier and we're here for you." Instead, they said: "Why are you back at work? You should be home with your baby."

That was 1979. Thirty-seven years later, we've made some headway in facilitating breastfeeding for working moms. Today, the judgment from yonder has a different stigma. Women are no longer deemed heartless for returning to work. Instead, they're deemed callous for not continuing to breastfeed, regardless. Rampaging breast milk diehards dole out advice, including the option to change the baby's schedule so *she sleeps* while *you work*, so you can be up all night nursing and playing with her when you get home. First of all, even if you believe this to be as ridiculous as I do *(When does Mom sleep, may I ask?)*, a small part of you feels inadequate for *not* doing this. Is breast milk *that* good that it is worth sacrificing your own mental and physical health, as well as that of your child? When we're sleep-deprived, scalding beverages are spilt, burners are left on, and babies are exposed to the misadventures of short-circuited brains.

If for any reason, you at some point realize that the benefits are not worth the pain or stress, it's acceptable—screw that: necessary—

for you to opt out of breastfeeding. Anyone who condemns you for this should open a wet-nurse pop-up shop and go milk themselves. Stock up on formula and, while you're at it, wine.

A Double-Edged Boob

Physically, everything was boobie-liscious for me. My breasts produced milk industriously (on most days), my nipples survived with very few bruises (though my boobs' elasticity—or what remains of it—is a different story), and my baby flawlessly latched onto them. Her stomach was a little sensitive, so I did have to play around with my diet and give up dairy...but as much as I love cheese, that was the easy part.

Emotionally, breastfeeding was the biggest challenge of motherhood I had to overcome.

You're told that this is such a beautiful experience—the best thing you can do for you *and* your baby. "It's *the* time to bond," I heard over and over again. No one told me that in actuality, I'd feel bound. That it would get lonely. That I would sometimes burst into tears after an hour of nursing because all I could do was sit there and stare at a wall.

Some women are able to wear their baby and cook dinner while they nurse. I needed a whole setup. I had a pillow on my lower back, a neck doughnut (which I highly recommend), a nursing pillow, and two cushions underneath one side or the other, depending on which boob she was sucking. This "fortress" bolstered my daughter up to an angle that helped her avoid gas and reflux. As she hungrily guzzled from my breast while I cursed myself for leaving my phone in the other room, I would idly wonder why on earth so many women just *love* breastfeeding.

It's not that I hated it. I really didn't. I mostly hated how *much* I had to do it.

For the first couple of months, my daughter needed to nurse as often as every forty-five minutes for at least one hour. I tried to stretch her feeding breaks to three hours because I wanted to have a life, but I received conflicting advice about resisting my daughter's cries.

"Sometimes babies just want the comfort of sucking," explained my mom-in-law. But the lactation consultant had warned me: "Don't let her be a snacker."

"I don't want her to be an emotional eater!" I would sob to my husband over our child's hungry wails—or "head banging" as we called it when she rooted. (The rooting reflex is when babies make sucking motions with their mouth as they move their head back and forth. To us, it looked like she was jamming to heavy metal.)

Time was slow and blurry those first three months after giving birth. Every day was Groundhog Day. *Wake. Sleep. Nurse. Burp. Shit. Change diaper. Pee. Change diaper. Cry. Wake. Sleep. Nurse. Burp. Shit. Change diaper. Pee. Change diaper. Wake. Sleep.*

Every night, I was summoned to my baby's room. I gave her the goods and then tiptoed out, like after a bad one-night stand, collecting shreds of clothing and modesty along my way. I felt like a milk whore. *Why buy the cow...?* I kept getting booby calls night after night, and I couldn't say no. I was the only one who could feed her.

My dear daughter *never* took a bottle. We once tried "starving her out" while I was at work to see if she would drink my breast milk from a bottle. Guess who lost that battle? She held out 'til I came home and nursed for two hours and forty-five minutes straight.

Being the ONLY source of nourishment for my daughter was extremely stressful. In the womb, her umbilical cord had been unusually short. Outside the womb, the metaphorical cord was just as tight.

PUSH TIPS for the Breastfeeding Mama

- Ask your nurse to put your baby on your chest as soon as she comes into this world—if possible, before they wash her and apply the eye drops. She'll be so alert, chances are she'll find your nipple and figure it out. Breastfeeding is instinctual for your baby.

- Take full advantage of the lactation consultant at the hospital if one's available. Ask her to teach you all the positions and help you both find the perfect latch. If your baby gets the latch just right out of the gate, your nipples may be spared a lot of agony.

- My lactation consultant told me to "present the breast" to my baby. Just like it sounds: You unleash it and place the areola in front of Baby's mouth. He can take it from there.

- Almost the entire areola needs to be inside the baby's mouth. If you have too much areola hanging out, your baby is just bruising your nipple and not getting as much milk per suck. Pull him away and re-latch.

- Your baby's mouth needs to look like a fish when attached to the nipple. Her upper and bottom lips shouldn't be tucked in; you should be able to see them.

- If the sucking hurts, it could be that you're blistered. But it could also mean that the latch is not right. Your boobs may still hurt if you're doing it correctly, but if you have bloody or incredibly butchered nipples, it may be a good idea to have someone inspect the latch; there may be room for improvement.

- Let Baby tell you when she's done nursing. It's rude to pull out—unless she falls asleep with your boob in her mouth. Then she's the one who needs a few etiquette pointers.

- Nipple cream or lanolin ointment is a must for your nipples. I applied Lansinoh HPA lanolin religiously after every nursing session and survived unscathed. If you dislike lanolin, I recommend Mama's Nipple Butter by Earth Mama Angel Baby.

- You need to feed your baby no matter what. Don't be afraid to supplement or switch to formula.

- Don't ever dilute your breast milk with water. This may cause brain swelling, which could lead to death.

- If there are no latching issues, try a bottle as early as possible. I still wonder if our baby would have learned to drink out of a bottle if it had been presented to her earlier than four weeks.

- Download the Kindle App on your phone, STAT. This palm-sized entertainment doesn't require two hands to operate. I devoured books while nursing with the help of my opposable thumb.

The Grass Is Always Greener

My friends who had a hard time producing enough milk seemed to spend a lot of time trying to churn it out. They committed to triple feeds (a merciless routine performed every feeding cycle, where you breastfeed for twenty minutes and then pump for twenty more while someone else feeds Baby previously pumped milk or formula); took Domperidone (a drug currently not approved for sale in the U.S. that is generally used to treat gastrointestinal disorders but has also been shown to increase prolactin, hence stimulating milk production); or spent a small fortune on supplements that claimed to boost their juice. I have to admit that if I'd had a low milk supply, butchered nipples, or latching issues, I wouldn't have tried as hard as they did.

But my friends who struggled with milk production seemed bent on doing the impossible to provide breast milk to their children. While I applauded their commitment, I envied that their babies could drink out of a bottle. For me this meant freedom. Little did I know that they felt just as trapped as I did—shackled to a machine or bound by the pressure they felt to breastfeed.

Grass. Is. Always. Greener.

In retrospect, it seems we all could've been happier if we had confronted our particular breastfeeding challenges, given it our best fight, and then graciously accepted defeat instead of letting it tear us apart. But at the time, I was frustrated at not having control over my baby's feeding preferences. It felt hard to play a good hand with the cards I'd been dealt.

How I Learned to Stop Sobbing and Love the Boob

By the end of the third month, my daughter and I had fallen into a rough routine. How did we get there? My iPhone Kindle, TV marathons, and honestly, throwing in the towel.

I finally stopped trying to put my daughter on a schedule that suited me and allowed her to nurse on demand, at least while on maternity leave and, after that, on weekends. I resigned myself to the Milking of Ivette García Dávila.

And this resignation soon turned into a realization—something most mothers know from the get-go: I was hers. I belonged to my daughter, breasts and all. Much more than she belonged to me.

Somewhere, somehow, the woman who wanted to stop breastfeeding at three months and pitied moms who seemed too attached to this process, fell in love with it. I fell in love with the ritual. With the closeness. With her sweet face and cute little dimpled hands pumping the uneven pruned breasts that I carried just for her in case she was hungry, tired, or just wanted comfort. I will forever miss this intimacy, now that it's gone.

Breast Is, in Most Cases, Best

Nutritionally speaking, this fact is indisputable. Only in rare instances, such as poor mother nutrition, prescribed medication, or medical illnesses, would formula be preferred over breast milk.

Breast milk contains disease-fighting antibodies and immune cells. These antibodies are important because babies don't start making their own 'til they're about six months old. Also, nutrients in human milk are bioavailable (easily absorbed by body). Breast milk contains oligosaccharides (a.k.a. simple sugars) that help fend off infection and host a healthy flora party in the gut. Tata juice also fluctuates in calorie content and flavor, providing the opportunity to expose your baby to a variety of tastes that could enhance his palate later in life. Additionally, breast milk provides essential fatty acids for brain growth,

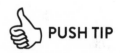 **PUSH TIP**

Pump the Vitamin D

The AAP advises that breastfed infants take a vitamin D supplement of 400 IU/day because breast milk contains only 25 IU of vitamin D per liter or less. Consult your doctor for a recommendation on infant-safe vitamin D drops.

along with prebiotics and proteins that support the immune and digestive systems (as do most formulas, by the way).

These benefits are widely celebrated. But I needed to know more. During my breastfeeding saga, I delved deeper into many claims about the cure-all effects of breast milk. I found some to be true, some to be false, some to be somewhere in between. Here's what I learned.

TRUTH OR STRETCH?
Debunking Some Tata-Juice Myths

#1 *Breast milk is a cure-all that protects your baby against disease*

True—except for the "all." Breast milk *does* provide immunity benefits, but it's not a panacea.

Your breast milk is specifically designed for your baby. It's built with germ-busting super-ingredients that respond to pathogens in your environment. Numerous studies have shown that stomach viruses, gastrointestinal infections, lower-respiratory illnesses, ear infections, and meningitis are less frequent in babies who are breastfed and are less severe when they do occur.

The main immunity shield that breast milk provides is a substance called secretory immonuglobulin A (IgA). Large amounts of this are present in colostrum, the first milk your body produces. This juice coats mucus membranes to prevent germs from invading your baby's intestines, nose, and throat.

Yet it's important to highlight that most of the antibodies that protect babies in early life are also acquired from the placenta during pregnancy and from the birth canal during vaginal birth. Also, once babies are exposed to other children and germs, there is very little that breast milk can do to keep them from getting sick. My breastfed daughter was sick for ten months straight after she started daycare. So was I.

#2 *Women shouldn't breastfeed while sick*

False. Most experts agree that unless a woman is taking medication that is incompatible with breastfeeding, it's not necessary for her to stop while she's ill. A mom can pass antibodies to her baby through her breast milk, which may help Baby counter the bug without necessarily catching it.

#3 *Breast milk will get your child into an Ivy League school*

It's true that breast milk helps support brain growth—though, of course, admittance to a particular college isn't guaranteed!

A 2016 study by Brigham and Women's Hospital shadowed 180 premature babies from birth to age seven and concluded that those who consumed predominately breast milk in the first twenty-eight days of life had higher IQs, working memory, motor function, and academic achievement. And that says something—a lot, actually. But many other influences—education, geography, parental involvement, social status...a little something called genetics—are also at play, which are hard to quantify scientifically, especially long-term.

Many experts agree that breastfeeding mothers generally have higher IQs and provide a more intellectual home environment than their formula-feeding sisters. When these observations are taken into account, the cause-effect relationship between breastfeeding and baby smarts becomes less clear.

#4 *Breast milk is free*

Ha. As Hanna said: "Only if a mother's time is worthless." And that's not even counting the boob job you'll need when your tits go belly down. In the words of a well-meaning breastfeeding veteran: "Just think of a balloon that gets blown up and then deflated. Over and over again."

For reference, the cost of feeding a baby formula for a year is estimated at about $2,000. That puts a value on my 829.5 hours at $2.41/hour. I can't even see the glass ceiling from that low.

#5 *Breastfeeding is convenient*

Often true, but the final judgment is subjective to each individual.

Breastfeeding can be incredibly practical. For Mom, it is convenient in that you don't have to get up, wash bottles, prepare "meals," remember to pack enough fixings while on the go, or even pump. (And if you're not pumping, your partner doesn't have to lift a finger. Maybe that's why they encourage it so much.) I loved popping out a boob and not having to pause the current TV marathon of choice.

However, in cases where it wasn't "socially acceptable," I often found myself huddled in a dirty bathroom stall or in the backseat of my car, wishing I could comfortably feed my baby out in the open—from a bottle *or* a boob.

To the prudes (including my husband) who don't like moms to nurse in public: If I do this all over again, I'm letting it all hang out. I hated leaving the room, the conversation, or the food on the table to go feed my child, for everyone else's sake.

#6 *Breastfeeding improves bonding*

Not necessarily.

We don't need an oxytocin release to fall in love with our babies—we bond with our babies in so many other ways. However, there *is* a sweet connection that can develop during breastfeeding. I really liked the feeling of being needed. Being the only person who could comfort my baby at certain times made me feel special in a way I'd never felt. When I analyzed this feeling, however, it didn't seem totally emotionally healthy. I fear that my own "bonding" bordered on codependence.

#7 *Best for Baby, best for Mom*

True, for the most part.

Some studies show that breastfeeding helps lower the risk of high blood pressure, diabetes, and cardiovascular disease in children. It may also help decrease the risk of uterine, ovarian, and breast cancers in moms. Amazingly, breastfeeding's protection against breast cancer builds up over time; that is, the duration of breastfeeding and the number of children who are fed. For every twelve months of breastfeeding (with just one child, or as the total period of time for several children), the risk of breast cancer decreases by 4.3 percent, compared to women who do not breastfeed.

However, you can also lose up to 5 percent of bone mass while breastfeeding, which can lead to osteoporosis later in life. It's unclear whether this is due to your baby's drawing up calcium or because your body is producing less estrogen, which is what helps your body absorb calcium. (Estrogen levels are decreased during breastfeeding to allow the release of prolactin, the hormone that stimulates milk production.)

#8 *Breastfeeding reduces risk of SIDS*

SIDS—sometimes known as "crib death"—stands for Sudden Infant Death Syndrome. This shit still scares the crap out of me, because to this day, SIDS remains a medical conundrum.

The answer: Probably. A meta-analysis noted that breastfeeding (both partial and exclusive) is associated with a 36 percent reduced risk of SIDS. A controlled case study also suggested that the positive effect of breastfeeding on SIDS rates is independent of the newborn's sleep position. However, the statistics that name breastfeeding as a reducing factor against SIDS tend to drop when other elements such as socioeconomic status and smoking are taken into account. However, there *is* a correlation between NOT breastfeeding and SIDS.

Two theories that link breastfeeding to SIDS prevention are:

○ Because SIDS appears to be linked to the inability to wake up from deep sleep, some experts think breastfed infants are less prone to die of SIDS because they sleep less soundly than formula-fed babies.

○ According to a study led by Associate Professor of Family Medicine at the University of Virginia, Dr. Fern Hauck, breastfed infants have fewer bouts of lower-respiratory infections, which are associated with vulnerability to SIDS.

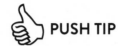 **PUSH TIP**

SIDS: Minimizing the Risk

In addition to breastfeeding, here are a few other recommendations to consider:

- Periodically check in on your sleeping baby or sleep in the same room with your baby, but not in the same bed.

- Lay your baby on his back to sleep.

- Stop swaddling as soon as Baby is able to roll onto his side or belly.

- Avoid putting pillows, bumpers, or stuffed animals in Baby's crib.

- Make sure your baby is not too hot by regulating the room's temperature and making sure he's not overclothed.

- Give your baby a pacifier when sleeping. Note: If breastfeeding, make sure a good nursing relationship has been established before introducing a pacifier.

#9 *Breastfeeding reduces risk of asthma, eczema, & allergies*

Inconclusive.

The somewhat plump skinny: A 2011 study by the European Lung Foundation concluded that feeding a baby breast milk exclusively for up to six months after birth could reduce the risk of asthma-related symptoms (wheezing and persistent phlegm) in early childhood.

Yet, another study conducted by Joanne M. Duncan and Malcolm R. Sears for the Firestone Institute for Respiratory Health at St. Joseph's Healthcare and McMaster University noted that the reduction in childhood wheezing could be the result of protecting against viral infections and that allergies and asthma at later ages could actually increase with breastfeeding. They also found that studies have "generally failed to demonstrate a protective effect of breastfeeding on outcomes of atopic dermatitis, allergic sensitization, wheezing, or asthma." Regarding eczema, the British Journal of Dermatology did a randomized study of over fifty thousand children from twenty-one countries and found no evidence that breastfeeding for four months or longer protects against eczema. However, these types of findings are wildly disputed. It seems nobody wants it proven that breast milk is not a get-out-of-jail-free card for every medical condition or disease.

Recent controversial research reveals growing evidence that breastfeeding exclusively for six months could actually put babies at risk of allergies (especially gluten), food aversion, iron deficiency, and even obesity. But this hasn't been proven or gained traction. This observation could be explained by the breastfeeding mother's diet and/or the absence of solids in babies' diets who are four months or older.

#10 *Breastfeeding is better than Weight Watchers*

Also inconclusive.

Some studies find that breastfeeding promotes weight loss, while others conclude that it doesn't.

Breastfeeding does make your uterus contract back to normal size. And it's a fact that your body burns calories producing milk (approximately 450/day), so you could lose weight. I did, and many other women do, too.

But that may take some self-discipline on top of the "supernatural" slimming benefits of breastfeeding. This is especially true because prolactin (the milk-producing hormone) is an appetite stimulant. So breastfeeding moms can end up eating more or making unhealthy choices. It's hard to make a salad when you're tied up to your baby;

meanwhile, chomping on potato chips requires only the use of one hand. We're also prone to be sedentary, as we can't really run that lap around the track while breastfeeding. Not to mention the time and energy breastfeeding steals from us.

If you do make the effort to exercise and eat healthy, it can be annoying when somebody assumes you got skinny due to breastfeeding. Make sure you take credit for that ass!

#11 *Breastfeeding prevents obesity in your child*

This is a bit of a stretch. While it doesn't prevent it, breastfeeding does provide "some level of protection against childhood obesity," according to a study conducted by the WHO. Others have arrived at similar conclusions. An editorial by Dr. William H. Dietz published in 2001 stated that children who were breastfed for at least seven months had a lower risk of being overweight than children who were breastfed three months or less.

But, again, one might argue that those kids who breastfed longer had parents who were more health-conscious or had some other attribute that played into this correlation.

#12 *Breastfeeding prevents pregnancy*

False. The odds are slighter, but what do you think Irish twins are?!

The University of Maryland Medical Center confirms that getting pregnant while breastfeeding can and does happen. Most breastfeeding moms experience lactation amenorrhea (LAM), which means they have little or no periods. This can lead them to falsely believe that they are not ovulating. If you're not looking for another baby, get on the mini-pill or shrink-wrap the perpetrator.

#13 *Breastfeeding reduces stress*

True, biologically speaking.

Numerous studies have found that breastfeeding promotes relaxation because your body secretes oxytocin. However, breastfeeding is only relaxing if you enjoy the experience, don't have work stress about nursing and/or pumping, and your milk supply doesn't cause you anxiety. That's a lot of ifs.

#14 *Breastfeeding delays menopause*

Maybe...and as someone with early menopause in her family, I'm psyched!

I found an awesome study by a Dr. M.D. Mazumdar, which I'll try to give you with a little bit of sugar. Because let's face it: This medical stuff is hard to swallow.

We are born with about two million follicles in our ovaries. By the time we're forty, this number has dwindled to eight thousand. Menopause happens when we run out of these follicles. During pregnancy, we stop menstruating for nine-plus months, which means we save some follicles. Ovulation is also "arrested" for about five to six months while we're breastfeeding, so it is likely that both pregnancy and breastfeeding could delay the onset of menopause.

However, it is important to make the distinction that even though you're not ovulating and menstruating, those follicles and ovaries are aging right along with you. So even though menopause may hit a little later, the quality of your eggs is not being preserved. Unlike a good cheddar, they do not get finer with age.

#15 *Your tits will go to shit*

I wish I had better news for you.

Not only are mine still disproportionate two years after giving birth, but my smaller right boob looks like a saggy testicle with a nipple on it. TMI?

BOTTOM LINE

Assuming you don't have a medical condition or take medication that is incompatible with breastfeeding, breast is best—but *only* if you're happy breastfeeding.

And if you can't or choose not to breastfeed, your baby will thrive with your truly unique mother's love and, yes, with formula. In a recent *I'm The One Pushing* podcast, I interviewed KPCC's *Morning Edition* host Alex Cohen, who shared an invaluable perspective she had gotten from another mom: "Go to a playground, look at the kids playing on the structure, and tell me who was nursed and who wasn't."

I'm a C-baby *and* a formula baby—can't you tell?

Love in the Time of Formula

This may shock you, but formula is not poison. The formula industry arguably self-inflicted this stigma back in the eighties when they marketed to low-income mothers, often providing free samples to get them hooked. Not armed with resources or proper education about formula usage, these mothers began mixing (and often diluting) the formula with questionable water sources, which led to serious repercussions and an ensuing scandal.

> "Formula is not talked about until you have to use it."
>
> —Lisa McGuire, Film Producer,
> Los Angeles, CA, Mother of One

But the truth is that formula was never a bad option. And these days, some organic brands are very close to the real thing.

Formula-feeding has many other perks, including that your baby will probably take in higher quantities of iron, vitamin D, and vitamin K (though iron in breast milk has a higher absorption rate). Possibly the most valuable benefit is that it gives Mom a wider range of motion after baby is born. She can be away for longer periods and be free from the hateful pump. Formula is the best option for many full-time working moms and/or single moms.

Outside of work and relationship situations, I know many other ladies who have opted for formula over breast milk—or at least embraced it along the way. Some went this route because breastfeeding was physically difficult for them. One friend simply couldn't abide the feeling of her baby sucking on her nipple; so she supplemented right away and stopped breastfeeding completely after three months when she returned to her desk. Her daughter is a bright, healthy, fierce little girl.

But if you've had your heart set on breastfeeding, feeding formula to your baby can be distressing. I know many strong women who have suffered this type of heartbreak. Barriers such as low milk production, or complications like mastitis or thrush can really throw a wrench into your plans. Or, if your baby is premature and/or spends time in the NICU (due to low birthweight, jaundice, etc.), she may need to be introduced to formula early on.

When difficulties with milk production arise, some moms become obsessed with making it happen and get frustrated with their bodies. If this happens, try to focus on what a wonderful thing your body *did* just do: It grew a baby! Supplementing with formula or switching over to it completely is the best option for many moms.

Wet Nurse, Anyone?

As an alternative to formula, you can source breast milk from another mom. I recommend procuring only from a regulated bank or a trusted relative or friend, as there is inherent risk involved, including salmonella contamination. Another cause for concern is that some unscrupulous sellers may dilute breast milk with water or cow's milk.

If you choose this option, also make sure to ask for proof of current blood tests that screen for HIV, syphilis, hepatitis, and human T-lymphotropic virus.

Nuzzling and feeding is a great bonding experience whether your baby's plugged in to a flesh nipple or a silicone one. Don't let a poor milk supply ruin your newborn motherhood experience. This time passes slowly, but it's still over before you know it.

What Is a Supplemental Nursing System?

A Supplemental Nursing System (SNS) is a device that simulates and stimulates breastfeeding.

The SNS is filled up with breast milk or formula, and liquids funnel through a capillary tube taped next to the nipple so baby suckles out of the nipple and the tube simultaneously.

The device was invented to incentivize a woman's breast milk supply and to help a baby learn to latch, but some moms who are unable to breastfeed have used it to mimic the act and foster the bonding it can provide.

IN SEARCH OF THE PERFECT FORMULA

It's hard to find high-quality formula, especially in the United States. I did a little research and polled my formula-feeding friends, and here's what I gleaned.

Most ladies in my mom's club recommend Baby's Only brand formula, citing that it has no glucose syrup, palm oil, or preservatives and that it comes in both a dairy and a lactose-free version. This formula is produced by a family-owned business in the U.S. Also, their formula with DHA/ARA doesn't use chemicals (hexane, in particular) to extract these essential fatty acids from its source. However, Baby's Only does contain taurine (see text box), apparently present in *all* formulas made in the U.S. But organic formulas should at least be free of the chemically produced taurine.

Some of my friends fed their babies exclusively European formula, claiming that dairy and cattle regulations are stricter overseas. They recommend Holle and HiPP.

Holle comes from grass-fed, organic, biodynamic sources (cow or goat milk versions available) and is free of soy, corn, and most synthetic ingredients found in mainstream formulas. Its Stage 1

Formula Ingredients to Consider Avoiding

Palm Oil: Many formulas include this to try to replicate breast milk's palmitic acid. However, palm oil isn't as readily absorbed by infants and may lead to decreased bone density.

Aluminum: Standard formulas—particularly hypoallergenic and soy-based ones—may contain up to forty times the aluminum found in breast milk. Aluminum may interfere with cellular activity and accumulate in the brain, resulting in brain dysfunction.

Carrageenan: This widely used thickening agent is derived from seaweed. Many deem it safe, but according to animal studies, carrageenan may lead to intestinal inflammation and colon tumors. This additive is banned from European infant formulas.

Taurine: The stuff they put in Red Bull. Enough said, right? But before you run away from it, know that natural taurine is a sulfur-containing amino acid that aids in metabolizing fats and is normally present in breast milk. However, man-made taurine is commonly manufactured via chemical synthesis and processed with carcinogenic sulfuric acid.

Soy: A plant high in estrogen, soy tends to be genetically modified and is usually produced with pollutants. Even lactose-based formulas may contain soy. Seek a brand that doesn't. If your baby is sensitive or intolerant to lactose, consider goat's milk or a formula that is both soy- and lactose-free. Also worth noting is that soy formulas often have a higher level of aluminum.

Sucrose, Maltodextrin, Glucose Syrup Solids, Brown Rice Syrup: These are all substances used to sweeten the "pot." If your baby has no sensitivities to it, lactose is the best sweetener you can find in formula.

If you have any further questions regarding quantities and/or ingredients' sources, contact your formula company's headquarters. They should have a dietitian on staff who can answer your inquiries.

Lebenswert also contains lactose instead of maltodextrin. However, Holle does contain palm oil.

So does HiPP, the other European formula heavyweight. HiPP is also made in accordance with Europe's organic, grass-fed regulations and it contains lactose and beneficial prebiotics. However, experts recommend using the ready-made version, as the powder variety tests high in aluminum.

If you're going Euro, procure ahead of time and buy in bulk, as shipping from overseas takes time. Most parents order from Organic Munchkin or Little World Organics.

Lastly, no matter what kind of formula fits your bill, always mix powder with filtered water and according to instructions.

Did I Say Breastfeeding Sucks? I Must Not Have Pumped Much.

I typed "what to buy to get ready for baby" into my search engine. A double breast pump popped up. Like a double rainbow, it blew my mind. I asked my friend Claire about it, whom I consider an expert on all things mom—or "mama," as she would say. She quickly explained: "You *have* to get the double one. I even got a bra that allows me to pump while doing dishes."

WTF.

I became haunted by this image. Myself pumping and barefoot, washing dishes in the kitchen. *Gosh, is this what's ahead?* We females are known for multitasking, but how about reading a book instead of scrubbing last night's casserole with two humiliating plastic cones extracting our female jizz?

WTF. WTF. WTFF.

I received a pump as a gift at my shower (from my boss, no less!). I left the Pandora's box unopened in a corner for months.

When I finally dared to open the contraption, I was aghast. It's 2017 and these things look like a prop from the movie *Frankenstein*. I'd rather be caught naked trying to open a jar of pickles (*Seinfeld*, anyone?) than with my nipples attached to a breast pump, ejaculating milk in a sequence of squirts that sound like a robot trying to piss a gallbladder stone.

We have Siri and self-driving cars, yet we can't figure out a *powerful* cordless breast pump or even (environment be damned) disposable cones so you don't have to wash them—or at least ones made out of silicone that comfortably conform to the shape of your breasts?

I'm personally offended that the pump industry hasn't made significant leaps in product development. It seems they're stuck in an *if-it-ain't-broke-don't-fix-it* mentality. Well, I'm here to tell them: It *needs* a-fixin'. In 2014, MIT Media hosted a hackathon entitled "Make the Breast Pump Not Suck"; some smart inventions were presented, but I'm not sure any of them provided a comfortable yet practical solution.

Breast Pumps: A History of Halted Progress

1854	First U.S. patent is issued for a breast pump.
1921	Edward Lasker produces a mechanical breast pump that imitates an infant's sucking action—a slight improvement on existing models.
1956	Einar Egnell publishes "Viewpoints on what happens mechanically in the female breast during various methods of milk collection."
1991	Medela, a Swiss company, introduces first consumer-grade electric-powered breast pump in the U.S.
1996	Medela quadruples sales by introducing the "swank" Pump In Style model.
2017	Medela Pump In Style Advanced with On-The-Go tote (or backpack) still retails for $191.02 to $299.99.

The Freemie seems to be going in the right direction by collecting hands-free directly into a concealable cup worn under your shirt. However, the reviews indicate that it has lower suction power than a traditional "horn pump" (the mainstream model that looks like you're sporting deer antlers on your tits) and that the valve is a PIA to clean. Others find it annoying because there's no timer to track pumping sessions, no measure indicating how much milk has been collected, and the collection cup doesn't double as a bottle or storage container. However, a friend of mine uses it and doesn't mind that it's slow, as she pumps while tied to her editing desk at work.

Most women pump so they can go back to work and still breastfeed. Yet, the most common reason women stop nursing altogether is because they go back to work. There are many deterrents to pumping at work.

If you share an office, you have to set time apart to hook yourself up to this human milking device while marooned in a supply closet with bad Internet reception. The time commitment is also stressful because you get behind on your work, when all you want to do is leave on time so you can go home to your human baby. I know a bunch of ladies who plug their devices into their cars and pump during their commutes to work to save time. That's award-worthy.

The hassles of pumping at work don't end there. After you're milked dry, you have to wash all the paraphernalia and store the goods appropriately. God forbid your precious milk spoil or spill. Thank God the lady at The Pump Station in Hollywood advised my friend (who then told me) that I could put all the gear in the fridge after each use and only wash it at the end of the day. This was face-saving advice. Who wants to see me washing my pump tubes in the office break room? In fact, nobody at work wants to know or hear anything in relation to your pumping. Even if they ask, they're being polite—trust me.

And that's just at work. If you're out and about, you have to tote a cooler and a portable electric or manual pump. And then you have to hide in a bathroom or behind a sunshade in your car covering your shameful breasts as you make a collection.

Another high percentage of women end up pumping because either their baby doesn't latch properly or they don't want to be beholden to an exclusive monogamous breastfeeding relationship with their babies. For twins, especially, pumping and formula can be a lifesaver.

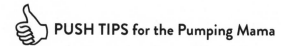 **PUSH TIPS for the Pumping Mama**

Very likely, you'll get mixed advice regarding when to start pumping. In general, as with everything, listen to your body.

If you're having trouble producing milk, pumping can stimulate your boobs into making it, so you may want to start immediately.

If you have no issues with milk production, the general consensus is to wait until you establish a nursing routine before you start building a bank, so that pumping won't interfere with feeding Baby—though you can always give him the pumped milk if your boobs are dry.

If you are an overproducer, you may want to pump anytime your breasts feel full, to avoid discomfort or, worse, a clogged duct.

Here are some more specific tips:

- **Your breasts will be fuller in the morning. If you can get "hooked up" first thing, you'll get a lot more milk per pump.**

- **If morning pumping isn't convenient, try it right before you go to bed, a few hours after your baby's taken her "last" drink for the evening. If she wakes up hungry during the night, you should have replenished by then. If not, send your partner in with a bottle so you can get some rest!**

- **If possible, set up a pump routine and stick to it. Your body will get used to producing extra milk at that time, and it will be easier for you to control leakage.**

- Hot showers helped me replenish supplies.

- Viewing pictures of your baby may speed up your "let-down" reflex. This is when milk starts releasing from your breast, usually about two minutes into nursing or pumping. To me, it felt like electric needles pricking my boobs.

- Consider pumping from only one breast while you're first building a bank. I did this if I knew she was close to nursing, so I would have one full breast for her.

- Don't fill a milk bag all the way to the top; contents will expand when frozen and spill over. And you *will* cry over spilled breast milk.

- When possible, pump directly into a bottle. It's one less thing to clean up.

- If you're going to pump a lot, invest in a pumping bustier.

- If you're an on-the-go gal, invest in a manual hand pump as well. You don't have to assemble it or plug it in.

- Store your milk in 1–2 ounce containers. This helps ensure you don't waste any milk if your baby doesn't drink a full bottle. An ice cube is about 1 ounce.

In case you can't tell, I really didn't take to pumping; but many women swear by it and even prefer it to breastfeeding. I, on the other hand, still mourn every minute I spent attached to the plastic breast ejaculator—all for naught. Every single bottle I tried to feed my daughter was never taken. It was a difficult time for me. So I turned to wine.

BUI: Breastfeeding Under the Influence

I'm half Cuban, half Puerto Rican. I love to drink. Drinking while breastfeeding is not something I recommend—but nor is it something I condemn.

Please read responsibly.

HOW MUCH IS REALLY SAFE FOR BABY?

Grandma's rule of thumb: Drink *while* you're nursing because it takes about one hour for the alcohol to make it to the breast milk.

She's not far off.

The AAP's Section on Breastfeeding states: "Ingestion of alcoholic beverages [while breastfeeding] should be minimized and limited to an occasional intake but no more than 0.5 g alcohol per kg body weight, which for a 60-kg [132-lb.] mother is approximately 2 oz. liquor, 8 oz. wine, or 2 beers. Nursing should take place 2 hours or longer after the alcohol intake to minimize its concentration in the ingested milk." Per Dr. Thomas Hale, who has performed extensive research on the effects of medication in mother's milk, states: "Mothers who ingest alcohol in moderate amounts can generally return to breastfeeding as soon as they feel neurologically normal" (*Medications and Mother's Milk,* 2012 Edition).

Famous blogger and international board-certified lactation consultant Kelly Bonyata from Kellymom.com agrees: "If you are sober enough to drive, you are sober enough to breastfeed," she says.

"Doctors don't know exactly how much alcohol goes into the milk," states Dr. Scott Cohen, author of *Eat, Sleep, Poop,* "but it is a very small amount, if any, and should not cause problems. With that said, you definitely shouldn't go on a drinking binge while you're nursing." Other experts agree, stating that only 2 percent of the alcohol consumed reaches Mom's blood and milk.

However, just like driving while intoxicated, drunk breastfeeding is not advisable. If you feel too drunk to drive, your milk alcohol level may not be safe either. If this happens, you—or better yet, a sober adult—can feed your baby previously pumped breast milk or formula. You will probably want to "pump and dump," too.

Pumping and dumping does not magically reset your alcohol levels back to sobriety. You pump to avoid clogged ducts and keep your milk supply regular. If you're at a party and feel like you're about to burst, go to the bathroom and jack off them boobs. You can save it if you feel sober enough to drive, or you can dump it if you're wasted (or perhaps someone may be interested in a Mother's Milk White Russian!).

Alternatively, you can invest in a pack of breast milk alcohol test strips. I've found mixed reviews from users—some women swear by them while others claim they're inaccurate or that the results seem to contradict expert's guidelines. I don't know anyone who has used them and they cost more than a decent bottle of wine, so I chose to buy the vino. (Not saying my choice is the smart one.)

I did most of my drinking after our daughter started to sleep through the night. That way, even if I had a few glasses of wine, I would be in the clear by the time she woke up in the morning.

I would be remiss if I did not to mention studies that suggest drinking more than one alcoholic beverage daily while breastfeeding could hinder your baby's sleep and affect her gross motor development. I didn't notice any irregularities in my daughter's sleep and, even though I don't know what her gross motor skills would be had I not drunk, she hit every milestone right along with her peers.

However, the truth is that drinking *could* affect your milk supply and your judgment, and those are good enough reasons not to drink.

But if you are going to try BUI, it may be worth experimenting during your longest breastfeeding break of the day (or night) to allow your boobs to fill back up and your milk's alcohol levels to drop. If you are breastfeeding exclusively (not formula-supplementing), you may want to plan ahead (pump and store), so that drinking doesn't interfere with feeding your baby—especially if you have issues with your milk supply. During the test run, you could also try pumping after a few drinks to test if the booze has affected your ejection "power."

Also, definitely consider your baby's age: A newborn has a teeny infant liver. A liver is more effective in detoxifying substances after a child is three months old.

CAN I USE BEER FOR A BOOST?

Another headline hitting the breast stands out there is that beer is a galactagogue: a substance that increases breast milk production by enhancing prolactin levels. My friend Claire swears that beer kept her milk a-comin'. It could be that she is just blessed with incredibly industrious, milky boobs. Or maybe she did find a particular beer that worked for her. It's worth giving it a responsible try to see how your boobs react.

But here's the catch: Even though barley (a grain widely used in beer) *is* a prolactin enhancer, alcohol itself reduces the body's prolactin levels. Alcohol can also inhibit oxytocin, which aids the milk ejection reflex. It has been proven that, overall, drinking alcohol reduces milk volume.

I occasionally had a beer during the day, and I did notice that some beers helped me produce more milk, while others...not so much. Guinness and Blue Moon worked for me. Pacifico didn't. But that's the one that did work for my friend Claire.

DRINK SMARTER, NOT HARDER

I have to confess to one drinking binge I had when our daughter was six months old. I was really shaken because I had just found out that a friend had killed himself. I was out to dinner with one of my best friends and we just went through that wine. And since it was the first time I had been drunk since before getting pregnant, it was a bad one.

I will regret drinking that much for the rest of my life. Though, *not* because of the alcohol content I may have arguably passed onto my child, but because of my lack of good sense.

My daughter didn't sleep through this particular night and woke up before sunrise. My husband brought her to me and I fell asleep while nursing her. A lot of people I know bed-share these days, but this was never for us for many reasons. Reason number one is that I'm an extremely sound sleeper. (Or was: It seems motherhood has stripped this ability from me.) I've slept through storms in a sailboat, small earthquakes, and large hurricanes. You can jump on the bed, graffiti my body, and fart on my face, and I won't wake up. Especially if I have been drinking. So that night, when she woke us up in the middle of the night, my judgment was clouded. And I was so tired. So I decided to nurse her in bed in our favored Dr. Sears–patented side-lying position. Normally I never fell asleep while nursing her in bed—my baby was a grunting machine and I could never really find a comfortable position. But this time I did. Hard.

I woke up late, and when I saw her sleeping so peacefully next to my hungover ass, haloed by the bright sun pouring in through the window, my heart almost stopped. I knew she could've suffocated while breastfeeding (a serious concern even for a sober mama who falls asleep while nursing) or that I could've rolled over onto her in my sleep. I was furious with myself.

I don't think I'll ever forgive myself for doing such an irresponsible thing. Even though it's incredibly embarrassing to admit what happened, I tell it as a cautionary tale to all drinking mamas out there. I've learned my lesson: Impaired judgment is the most important reason not to drink while breastfeeding or while being the responsible parent-in-charge.

Since then, my husband and I take turns being "on duty." You can't ever make the same mistake twice; otherwise, it's a choice, right?

THE *BABY,* THE *BOSS,* THE *HOME,* & *YOUR LOVER*

Juggling Life While Exclusively Breastfeeding

I PASSED THE BOX OF TISSUES to the new mother sitting across my desk with a hospital-grade pump resting between her legs. Amidst sobs, she mewled a few sounds that when pieced together spelled out that she wasn't ready to be back at work. This was her third day at the office, and her baby was turning four months.

"I just miss her so much," she repeated.

I did my best to appear sympathetic, but I'd take on hysterical infant triplets any day over one crying adult.

Based on the number of women who have spilt tears in my office, you would guess I'm either a therapist, a social worker at a women's shelter, or a funeral director. At the time, I was actually the Executive Vice President of a reality TV casting company; I can assure you the drama extends beyond the set. This particular gal had good reason to weep, though. Going back to work after having a baby is tough stuff.

Yet, as I sat there trying to comfort her, all I could think was: *How come I never really felt like this? Is there something wrong with me?* After my own maternity leave, I was high-fiving my brain the minute I was back at my desk.

State of the Union: Maternity Leave

I went back to work exactly three months and three days after our daughter was born. In the U.S., employers give new moms anywhere from zero to six months of maternity leave, sometimes paid, often not. Most parents end up taking accrued vacation and sick days to patch together a "family leave."

Maternity Leave Laws

If you live in California, New Jersey, or Rhode Island, you may be eligible to collect disability during the last couple of weeks of your pregnancy and/or Paid Family Leave (PFL) benefits after your baby is born or adopted. (New York passed the Paid Leave Benefits Law in 2016 and it will become effective in January 2018.)

In the state of California, you get ten to twelve weeks of paid disability and family leave combined, depending on whether you delivered vaginally or had a C-section. You can choose to start your disability benefits prior to delivery or wait until D-day. The California PFL alone covers up to six weeks and the benefit amount is approximately 55 percent of your weekly wage.

A good thing to know is that you can defer PFL and collect it any time in the first year after Baby is born. PFL benefits any employee who needs to care for a relative, not just infants, and your co-parent is also eligible to collect.

For more information:

- Go to your state's employment development department (EDD).

- Check out nationalpartnership.org.

- Visit the National Conference of State Legislatures page on State Family and Medical Leave Laws (ncsl.org/research/labor-and-employment/state-family-and-medical-leave-laws.aspx).

Many feel that the U.S. doesn't support a proper maternity or paternity leave compared to other countries. These feelings seem justified, as we are the only industrialized nation without mandatory federal paid leave for new families. About 40 percent of workers in the U.S. aren't even covered by the 1993 Family and Medical Leave Act, which protects a new parent's job for twelve weeks after birth or adoption without promise of pay. Thankfully, some avant-garde states do allow benefits for Paid Family Leave (PFL).

Although my employer did not provide any maternity leave benefits whatsoever, I was lucky to live in one of three states that issues disability and family leave assistance. I ended up using three sick days before pushing, and afterwards claiming my disability benefits until they ran out and rolled into PFL. I rounded out my "parental sabbatical" with two weeks of unpaid leave. I wanted to have a full three months with my baby.

By the end of that time, I was ready to get back in the saddle. Of course, I had no idea how hard it would be to ride that bull. It's character-building to say the least.

Milked Dry

Rather than sorrow over my maternity leave ending, I felt stress— emotional, physical, and financial. My challenges were entirely different from those of my friends who suffered feeling estranged from their babies. I didn't miss my baby—I was nursing her every three hours!

As you well know, my daughter never took a bottle—any bottle. And we tested every nipple on the market, so please stop asking. We also tried occupational therapy, starving her out, the bait and switch...nothing worked. It turns out her issue wasn't behavioral but physical—she couldn't suck on a pacifier, either. (But she wasn't tongue-tied, so a frenotomy or a frenectomy [snipping or revising the frenulum] wouldn't have helped.) Because of this, in order for me to bring home some bacon *and* sustain our daughter, we had to hire a nanny who could bring her into my office to feed off my fountain of breasts.

I was lucky to work for a company that allowed me to nurse at work. I was permitted to turn a closet into a "nursery," fully amenitized with a skylight, a changing table, and a hard drive bank emitting electromagnetic fields.

Yet, even in the most supportive work environment, it's extremely hard to keep up with breastfeeding once you return to your post. "To follow a doctor's orders, a woman who returns to work twelve weeks after childbirth has to find a way to feed her baby her own milk for another nine months," Jill Lepore stated in her astute 2009 "Baby Food" article in *The New Yorker*. For most mothers this means pumping; in my case, this meant a (literally) draining work/nursing schedule. When mothers go back to work, "the nation suffers," as she put it, "from a Human Milk Gap."

While the nation was suffering from a Human Milk Gap, my daughter was drinking it from the source. My daughter's inability to drink out of a bottle forced me into a crazy, almost impossible routine. I worked from home in the mornings from 5:30 to 10:00 a.m. to "fill her up." Then I would go to the office; work my ass off 'til my daughter arrived ready to nurse; use up whatever lunch break I could hoard that day (in my industry, you eat in front of your computer) to play with her; and then the nanny would take her to the park or on a walk through seedy Hollywood while I tried to work instead of worrying about all the perils they could encounter out there with all the fake superheroes and real weirdoes on the Boulevard.

When they got back safe and sound around 3:00 p.m., I would thank the heavens and squeeze in another feed. At 5:59 p.m., I would rush my boobs home so my daughter could breastfeed two more times before going down for the night. If I was fortunate, she would sleep 'til dawn, when she would eagerly seize the boobs again. And again. And again.

Any questions so far about why I hated my breastfeeding routine during this time?

Every work/nurse day was an updated version of my former Groundhog Day hell. When she napped, I worked from my laptop. When she nursed, I worked from my iPhone. At the office, I nursed shamelessly during all-female meetings. While nursing my baby to sleep, I read and typed long responses with my one free thumb to end-of-day reports from various teams I managed. When she was finally in her crib—and if I was lucky enough to be done with work—I had about an hour to cook and feed my husband and me (or chow on some takout) before passing the fuck out, just to live the same day all over again. I was stuck in a circle of Dante's Inferno, and it wasn't divine.

Dropping the Ball

This routine was killing me softly and embittering me swiftly. The day my daughter turned one, I felt I had to throw in one of the balls I was juggling. So I chose to drop the soul-crushing ball of hell: my job. And not only because of my demanding schedule.

The moment I became a mom, my professional goals shifted.

Becoming a mother has made me hyperaware of the short time we are here on this world, I wrote in my resignation letter to my boss, *and if I were to die tomorrow, I don't want this to be the only professional thing I accomplished.*

I wanted to seek more.

And yet...

My boss, who is also a woman, called a meeting on my last day to announce to the staff that I was leaving to become "a better mommy and a better wife." Even though she probably didn't mean it the way it sounded (just to give her the benefit of the doubt), I've never been so humiliated in my entire professional life.

And let me tell you: I've been through it all. I've stocked tampons in Mary Louise Parker's trailer; I've been told by a former boss who is a top Hollywood producer: "Of course I know who you are: you're Ivette with the great ass"; I've worked for an Academy Award-winning director who blamed me for his not taking his vitamins because I had gotten him an unsightly pillbox; I've been yelled at by a two-bit producer amidst a prison scene with a hundred-plus mean-looking extras on a Steven Segal movie set; I popped an Airborne fizzy tablet in my mouth like it was an Altoid in front of Kevin Nealon (he never let me live that down); I even (poorly) hit on Ryan Gosling once to help a friend in need.

Needless to say, I'm not easily embarrassed, shaken, or stirred. I've got that thick skin people say you need to have in order to "make it."

Yet, with just one sentence, my boss, my mentor, my friend—an "enlightened" woman who had allowed me to breastfeed at work—reduced my contributions to the company to microbial levels and made me feel like a cold, flat forgotten popcorn kernel in the dark corner of an insalubrious theater next to ten-year-old gum. It took every ounce of my self-control to not bawl uncontrollably like that new mom in my office who wasn't ready to be back at work. I barely made it to my car. I really took that comment to heart and, to this day, it pains me to relive it.

Telling my co-workers that I was leaving to be "better" at motherhood and wifehood was not only an insult to me, but to all womankind. It reinforced the regressive notion that women can't do it all—or at least not *well*.

A Mother in the Modern World

It's still shocking to me that our "modern" society doesn't support women who strive to juggle a career and motherhood, or as some say, "have it all." We need to speak up—scream loudly, really—for our families, employers, and government to better support breadwinning parents.

That said, it's equally outrageous that this same society condescends to women who choose to exclusively raise children and run the home.

We're all mothers, and it would be nice to have each others' backs. Yet, we struggle to find appropriate terms for any kind of mom, paycheck-earning or not.

Let's run through the gamut:

"Stay-at-Home Mom": Really, you just stay at home—as if on house arrest?

"At-Home Mom": Mom is not a mom outside the home. Just inside.

"Homemaker": So, only those without jobs make a home?

"Working Mom": Because women without jobs don't work as hard? And let's not even start on why nobody calls a man a working dad.

"Full-Time Mom": And employed moms aren't? Show me where the punch clock is, please!

"Domestic Engineer": I like that it tries, but it takes the heart out of it.

Now, I don't think these terms are trying to be offensive... it's just really hard to come up with a fair term for what we do. In fact, the most appropriate term for all moms might be "Do-It-All Goddesses"—but I'm reserving that one for all the single mamas out there.

In an attempt to find a "label" for the main kinds of mothers, I've come up with some terminology. For this book's purposes, moms whose primary time commitment is taking care of their children and home shall be dubbed "Home-Runner Moms." Moms who have other time-consuming commitments, such as a job, shall be referred to as "Breadwinner Moms." And as aforementioned, single moms shall be "Do-It-All Goddesses." Moms who are students or active volunteers in their communities can probably find a little of themselves in each category. In fact, all mom functions overlap, because we're really that good at multitasking.

Like most jobs, all mom positions come with perks and setbacks.

WANTED: HOME-RUNNER MOM

Parenting is hard work, and people who are solely devoted to this duty deserve utmost admiration and respect.

As the sole caregiver for our daughter while my husband was out of the country, I was ready to pluck every single strand of hair out of my head, one by one. I had moments of pure bliss that only a child can give you, but they were interspersed with moments of disarray, frustration, boredom, and exhaustion. Raising children is one of the most challenging, magnanimous, and rewarding careers out there.

My grandmother Mamá Gloria happily hid her Bachelor of Science degree inside the closet and went on to raise five amazing women—all creative, autonomous professionals—and seven adoring grandchildren. Every time I think of Mamá Gloria, I think of the Ralph Waldo Emerson quote on my fridge:

> *To laugh often and much;*
> *to win the respect of intelligent people*
> *and the affection of children;*
> *to earn the appreciation of honest critics*
> *and endure the betrayal of false friends;*
> *to appreciate beauty; to find the best in others;*
> *to leave the world a bit better, whether by a healthy child,*
> *a garden patch, or a redeemed social condition;*
> *to know even one life has breathed easier because you have lived.*
> *This is to have succeeded.*

Hands down, Mamá Gloria triumphed.

I wish she were still around to ask if she has any major regrets about choosing to be a Home-Runner. I'm willing to bet she'd say no. When I worry that maybe she sacrificed her own needs, I must only think of her lush garden. She genuinely loved caring for things. She was giving, selfless, and full of sass.

Mamá Gloria was a true feminist and matriarch. Choosing to focus all of your energy on your children and home doesn't make you any less intelligent or influential than your peers. Your legacy is likely to live through many generations. Just be sure to take the time to nourish yourself, too. It's very easy to forget about you. Don't. Get help with the kids, because you'll need it, and take time to exercise, to do your hair, to read a book...take at *least* one hour every day JUST FOR YOU. Your family will reap the benefits of a happy mom.

WANTED: BREADWINNER MOM

The desire to pursue a vocation can very well be intellectual rather than just financial. Loving and excelling at being a mother doesn't mean you have to let go of your other aspirations. In fact, pursuing your dreams can be a great example for children. A recent study by Harvard University concluded that daughters of moms who work are likely to earn more money in the workplace and sons are likely to be family-oriented.

Unfortunately, most Breadwinner Moms still end up doing the majority of the home-running too. I was one of them. When I was working, I still felt like I had to do it all on top of my job, including finding time to love, feed, play, and read to my sweet baby girl. I ran the shit out of the household with the help of Amazon Subscribe and Save. I grocery shopped every week to make sure we were stocked up on organic crap. I managed to cook something edible a few times a week. I kept up to date with our daughter's wellness and physical therapy visits for torticollis and bottle-latching issues. I tracked my daughter's growth and vaccine chart. I scheduled play dates. I sent timely thank-you notes. I even managed to look halfway fuckable half the time. The other half, I looked like a malnourished, veiny, scraggly-haired lizard woman.

As Belinda Phipps, chair of the Fawcett Society for women's equality, said: "Women are still doing it all, not having it all" (*The Guardian,* June 2015). During this stage of my life, the one thing I never found time for was me. It's hard to find that hour for you, but singing to your favorite album on a long commute, a lunch away from your desk, even sneaking in a mani/pedi with a work friend can do wonders for your soul. Fit it in somewhere, somehow. And take a couple of hours to yourself during weekends. No guilt allowed. You deserve it.

WANTED: DO-IT-ALL GODDESS

Some moms choose or end up being solely in charge of all the financial, care-giving, and domestic duties that are required to raise a child and keep a cozy roof over his head. So they end up being the sole Breadwinners *and* Home-Runners. It takes a special kind of person to shoulder all of this with grace.

I have two friends who became moms through IUI and don't have co-parents. They're rock stars in my book, and they've taught me to be better at accepting help. If I ask them, "Can I watch your kid while you go get something to eat?", they're out the door before I'm even done with the question. They remind me that it does take a village and that having a supportive community is invaluable to any mother.

TO EACH MOM HER OWN

If you are torn between whether to be a Breadwinner or a Home-Runner Mom, a lot of logistics may factor in.

The decision to go back to work may be based on finances, as your paycheck may offset the cost of help. If you want a career, it may be worth it to just break even until your kid is in school. It's hard to pick up where you left off after five years.

Conversely, if you want to stay at home, your household may suffer from the loss of your income.

Working a job from home sounds convenient, but it's tricky. I've done it and I've found that I either shortchange my work or my daughter, or both. I've also found that it's impossible to do without using a television as a babysitter or hiring a nanny. At which point, I've wondered: *Wouldn't she be better off at daycare? So much cheaper than a nanny, too.* (Which is why she now goes to a place with trained caregivers.)

There are many important things to consider during this next stage, and yes, if you have a partner, they may have a say in your decision.

No matter what you decide, don't make the same mistake I did. I put everyone else first: baby, boss, husband, even my parents. And I burned the fuck out.

Whether you are a Breadwinner, a Home-Runner, a Do-It-All, or something in between, really strive to do what your heart sings. Aim to be the "Have-It-All" Mom.

Listening to my heart has always led me to where I want to be. But I relearned this after ignoring my heart for so long, lured by the sound of money hitting my bank account. *Cha-ching!*

In Pursuit of Happiness

My job paid well, but it was demanding. My boss and I co-managed a staff of twenty-five-plus and helped oversee numerous casting projects on our slate to ensure they were meeting our (very) high standards and our clients' (many) demands. Somewhere along the line, my work became less and less creative and more and more mind-numbing. My career in reality television and my job requirements became unbearable. I was in emotional limbo and at the threshold of joyless. I felt like my life was playing out on a TV in purgatory and I was just staring at it, waiting to be summoned. Then I realized that I was still alive and nobody was gonna call my name. So I called it.

I asked myself hard questions: *Is this the legacy I want to leave behind: managing adults who put people on reality shows? Reassuring grown-up clients that we can find thirty-something-year-old cougars (!!!) who are DTF* on television?*

(* = Down To Fuck)

The answer was simple: No.

If I had loved my job and what we were doing as a company, I would've stayed. I find managing twenty-five adults much easier than wrangling my infinitely beloved daughter. But I didn't want to wake up in twenty years financially stable but with a drawer full of broken dreams. So instead of staying focused on a safe career with a steady paycheck, I became driven to pursue the thing that has always made me happy: writing.

Having a baby made me remember that life is as precious as it is short. I didn't want to throw it away on a job that made me feel "icky" about myself. Now that I had fulfilled my lifelong dream of becoming a mom, it was time to pursue the other thing in life that made me feel alive.

But I knew this choice came with great monetary sacrifice and that I had to budget accordingly.

Luckily, I had worked my ass off after grad school, paid off my car and student loans, and had managed to save a little dough. I also knew I could pick up freelance casting work here and there. So I took the plunge.

Sometimes the freelance gigs don't add up and I struggle to pay the bills, but I hang in there knowing (or at least hoping) that working extra hard to pursue my dream job will pay off in the end. And if I fail, at least I sank while enjoying the swim.

I believe the secret to being happy and successful lies in the old cliché (I told ya I loved 'em!): "You have to do what you love and love what you do." Whether that's childrearing. or being a wife, a trapeze artist, a litigator, a sought-after nipple piercer, a fearless whale rider, or all of the above.

I didn't leave my job to become a better mommy and a better wife. I left it to pursue happiness. Which I guess, in the end, will make me "a better mommy and a better wife."

But only I can say that.

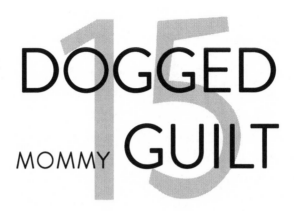

DOGGED

MOMMY GUILT

Bite It Before It Bites You

I WAS BITTEN by a Doberman pinscher named Hitler when I was twelve years old. (Actually, I recently discovered that his name was Hunty, but I've always remembered it as Hitler because that's how much I hated that SOB.) Anyway, needless to say, I'm a cat girl. My daughter, on the other hand, is a dog girl. When a dog is in range, my child becomes a magnetic force that pulls everything on her wake (me) towards the damn pup. I dread it every time, because it forces me to confront fears I'm not ready to overcome. Especially after what happened today at the market.

At our neighborhood farmers' market, people leave their dogs tied to posts unattended in a grassy area where kids like to jam to live reggae versions of classics such as "Wheels on the Bus." When my daughter took interest in a few unchaperoned dogs, I was able to redirect her—except when I wasn't.

She was an irresistible snow-white ball of fluff with long ears. Not too big, not too small—she seemed just right. My little girl tried to run to her, but I gently pinned her in place while I looked around for an owner. If he was around, he didn't indicate any interest in saying hello.

This cute thing was much different from the dog that bit me. This white dog was as tall as my mom's knee-high socks. Hunty had been statuesque. I had wanted to pet him, too, but the damn dog bit my hand when I tried. He was quick. His owner immediately pulled him off me before he had a chance to damage any nerves or bones. My hand was very lucky. My psyche was not.

Whenever I'm near a dog I don't know, a cloud of dread fills my chest, crushing my breath. When I try to fight it, a new layer of terror cloaks me, of fear that the dog can smell the fear. This is what I go through every time I see a new dog. I didn't want to pass this phobia on to my daughter. So like any parent who wants her child to explore the world, I took a calculated risk.

I pushed through my own issues, tucked my daughter behind me, and circumspectly approached the pooch. I extended my hand to the dog's nose, and it graciously let me pet it. We had a good time for a few minutes before I let my daughter come a few inches closer. She was dying to lean in to give the doggie a "kissie." She had just learned to "kiss" and loved kissing boys, dogs, and most recently, the phone when her daddy appeared on FaceTime. He was in Germany on business. I was home alone with this kid.

We get some *"awwws"* from the crowd, because it's so darn cute when a baby befriends a dog. I felt encouraged. We continued to cautiously court our four-legged friend. Until the little thing snapped at my daughter, just an inch away from her supple cheeks. I yanked her away and held her so tightly that I scared her even more.

In all honesty, I don't think the dog would've bitten her. He was likely just warning us that we were invading his space. But it scared the shit out of me nonetheless.

My daughter recovered more quickly than I did. Being the loving, trusting, and brave soul that she is, she was eager to say hello again in a few short minutes. I, on the other hand, wanted to commit a cold-blooded canine crime.

Instead, I clutched on to my baby and moved towards a mother who sat nearby with her own daughter. I was fishing for sympathy in the eye of an emotional storm, but the other mother didn't bother to look up, nor ask if we were okay. What she did do was proceed to tell her daughter loud enough that I could hear: "That's why we don't pet stranger dogs." I was wrong to think there were only four-legged bitches at the market that day.

I walked away from them and sat at a kids' table, rocking my daughter more for my own sake than hers. I felt a full-on bawling session brewing and I got us out of there before it erupted. I passed strangers, clenching my quivering jaw, thankful for the cheap pair of sunglasses I had "borrowed" from one of my sisters during my last trip to Puerto Rico.

Tears washed my face as I pushed the stroller on the walk home. I wept out of fear, relief, love, and embarrassment, but most importantly, out of guilt. I was inconsolable because I had taken a chance against my better judgment. I had let my child's strong will and my want for her instant gratification combined with my fear of her inheriting my baggage (which was now baggage on top of baggage)—win over. And I had failed her.

What if that dog had bitten her face? Her sweet cheeks, her two-tooth smile. What if that dog had given her a scar that made her resent me for the rest of her life?

When we finally got home, I sobbed on my baby's shoulder for the first time in her life. I felt incapable of keeping her happy, healthy, and safe. That judging mother at the farmers' market had made it worse because she had said out loud the same harsh judgment I was inflicting upon myself. But was she any different from me? I had secretly judged my own friends for their parenting decisions—things like feeding their kids too much meat or no meat at all. Most shamefully, I had also resented my own loving mother for so long. Like most women out there, I could write a book entitled *Mommy Issues: It's All Her Fault.*

The Blame Game

I have blamed (and judged) my mother for over twenty years because she didn't pick herself back up fast enough after my parents' divorce. Instead, she spent a year drinking scotch on the couch listening to the same songs over and over while I tried my best to look after my younger sisters. I expected my mom to be stronger than that, but she succumbed to depression when I needed her to keep her wits, to be there for us, to keep our home happy and running. I say that as if she had a choice. But back then I didn't know what I know now about depression. She was drowning, but I wanted her to be *my* version of the perfect mom. So, instead of throwing her a life jacket, little by little, I unraveled. In the span of four years, I went from being a pretty good kid who attended Catholic youth groups to being a runaway teen.

I started making wrong turns in the eighth grade, right after the divorce. Guys started to notice me because I lost a bunch of weight, and all of the sudden, I went from being Ms. Piggy to being Ms. Cute. I liked the attention. At this age, kids start dating, drinking, and smoking. Since nobody stopped me from doing any of this (in fact, I manipulated my mom into buying me booze and cigarettes), I kept going. I got sent to school after school, where I would fall in with the rebellious cliques 'til it was time to start over somewhere else. I got in trouble so many times, I was sure the world was wrong and I was right. I was contemptuously deaf to sensible advice. I wouldn't have even listened to my own adult self if time travel were an option. At that point, the only thing that could set me straight was to hit rock bottom. And that, I did.

After two boarding school attempts, I was placed to live with some distant relatives. But after breaking one too many rules, I was kicked out of their house, too. No one seemed able or willing to deal with me. *No one cares,* I thought. *I'm not important enough.*

I was so angry that I cashed a blank check and jumped on a plane bound for the Dominican Republic. I thought that since the

DR wasn't an American territory, my parents couldn't get to me there. My dad found my rental car (I had previously managed to destroy two cars we owned) in the airport lot, with a quarter pound of marijuana in it and my name graffiti'ed in blue ink over the vinyl seat, the "i" in Ivette topped with a heart. To my teenage self, it was the fuck-you of all fuck-yous. To my adult self, it was a cry for help.

When my mother heard I'd left the country, she threw an ashtray she had saved from her honeymoon onto the balcony floor. My best friend, who ratted me out after giving me all of five dollars to run away, witnessed the whole thing. She told me it shattered in so many pieces that shards of glass would be found on that balcony for decades to come. Little reminders of what used to be whole.

Meanwhile, I had found a place to live in the DR with some friends of friends. They put me up in a little girl's room that was pink and dizzyingly frilly—I felt like I was Barbie living in a Dominican Dreamhouse. Until the night I woke up on that twin bed with one of the "Ken's" who lived there standing over me, jacking off.

I ran away from him and locked myself in a bathroom. The guy pounded on the door, begging for forgiveness. Mainly because he was afraid I would tell his girlfriend, not because of what he'd done to me.

Now, I had fooled around with boys before; so even though I hadn't gone all the way, I knew how to handle myself. But awakening to an unknown one-eyed purple monster is nothing short of traumatic, no matter how tough you think you are. It would be jarring today at almost forty; imagine it happening to your sixteen-year-old self. Or worse yet, to your daughter.

It was on that bathroom floor in the Dominican Republic after one long month of being gone that I realized that by trying to punish my parents, I was really hurting myself. I decided I needed to come home. Get a high school diploma and move on with my life. At that young age, I understood that I alone had put myself in harm's way and that I could eventually ruin my life.

However, it wasn't until the moment I held my own daughter twenty years later after almost getting her bitten by a dog that I truly understood the relief, embarrassment, and guilt my parents must've felt when I came back home, thankfully unharmed. Actually, I'm sure my dad was worried sick, but I think moms are more prone to self-blame than dads (hence, the coining of the phrase "mommy guilt"). And for some fucked-up reason, as though it's encrypted in our DNA, some of us are also quicker to blame *and* judge our mothers and ourselves.

Standing in my mom's shoes, having failed my own daughter, I realized I had to stop blaming and judging my mother. I could now empathize with her. How she must have lain awake at night scared shitless of what could happen to me, unable to protect me. Helpless. Frustrated that she didn't have the tools to understand and stop me from doing bad shit. And then feeling relieved and grateful when I came home relatively in one piece. Yet overwhelmed with guilt over the way things turned out—over the things that could've been and never will. Yeah, my rebel bug had been exacerbated by my family's circumstances, but I now recognize how limited we parents really are in shaping our kids' destinies and how powerless we are against their wills and the world's. Not to mention that to err is simply parental.

Deciding to stop blaming my mom didn't magically eradicate my mommy issues, but it did land us on equal ground. It helped me see that we will all inevitably make mistakes with our own children and that they will blame us for them and that we will forever feel guilty about them.

Unless we stop the cycle.

Guilt: Do Not Recycle

Even those of us with great parents seem to find ways they fucked us up—or at least ways we would be better adults if they had done something differently. This feeling compelled me to try to one-up my mom in the art of motherhood.

In becoming a mom, I felt the pressure to live up to an ideal I had set for myself, eschewing the laundry list of shit for which I'd judged every parent I'd ever known, and drawing from all the seemingly "perfect" ones I'd encountered, real *and* fictional. This quixotic quest for perfection is to blame for the overwhelming guilt I feel when I fall short of my own hard-to-meet expectations and let my daughter pet unfamiliar, grumpy fluffy dogs when I know better.

Because of my own mommy issues and my desire to be better than my mom, I now felt extra terrible for having made a mistake with my daughter. I had set myself up to be above and beyond my own mother's qualifications and I had fallen short. At that moment, it was as though a fucked-up yin and yang symbol of "Mommy Judgment" and "Mommy Guilt" materialized before my eyes. I realized then that one couldn't exist without the other, and that they were both rooted in an unrealistic ideal of perfection. The judgment/guilt cycle thrives on the self-blame we feel—and dole out—over not being "the perfect mom."

As I cried hysterically on my daughter's shoulder, judging myself for failing my own ideals of maternal perfection, I felt compassion for the heartbroken woman my mom once was. Blaming ourselves (and our moms) is what moms (and daughters) do best. And we let that guilt gnaw at us like a dog with a bone.

My mom probably blamed herself for losing my dad (not being the perfect wife) and for not being strong for us (not being the perfect mom). She tried the best she could to pull herself together after the man she'd loved for eighteen years fell out of love with her—and she did. But it took her a while to get there. And who was I to judge or restrict the amount of time she was allowed to mourn the loss of her husband? A teenage brat, that's who.

If I couldn't be the perfect mom I wished to be, how the hell could I expect my mom to be the mom I wanted her to be?

I certainly hope it doesn't take my daughter thirty-seven years and motherhood incarnate to realize that no mom is perfect. And that an imperfect mother is not an incompetent or unloving mother.

Most importantly, I want my daughter to learn the art of forgiving herself after making a mistake, and be able to pick herself back up. If she masters this craft, then guilt may not bite her. She may even grow up to have fewer mommy issues than me (dare I hope?).

But first, I need her to understand the truth behind Martha.

Debunking the Marth

I'd love to ask Martha Stewart not how, but *why,* does she make it all look so elegant, serene, and clean? Why does she perpetuate the idea that a mom and her sweater can always be composed and coiffed, have manicured green thumbs, and be synonymous with a picture-perfect home? I would love to see Martha Stewart with banana matted in her unbrushed hair, attempting to scramble an egg in a half-washed pot while trying to keep a toddler from pulling down her scruffy pajama pants. I want to see her choosing to let her daughter watch yet another episode of *Sesame Street* because she simply doesn't have the energy or the desire to pretend-drink more tea. I want to see her being human.

Do you know how much judgment/guilt I have endured because of Martha Fucking Stewart? She's a businesswoman and a damn good one at that. Why? Because she figured out how to sell an illusion.

But that's all it is: a carefully produced and decorated mirage. You may be able to follow her snickerdoodle cupcake recipe, but you'll never be Martha Stewart. Because not even Martha Stewart is Martha Stewart.

Yet, I so wanted my mom to be like her.

But my mom has never had a garden. She has a hard time paying her bills on time. She toes the hoarder line. She talks constantly about her health issues yet does little to correct the behavior creating them. She always has an improvement plan that keeps being postponed. She still acts like a kid. And, as her daughter, I wish I didn't always have to be the adult. But just like every other imperfect mother out there, she deserves to be absolved of the "crime" of not living up to her daughter's expectations. This mommy judgment disease I'd contracted needed a cure before I ruined my own daughter. Had I forgotten all the beautiful and meaningful things my mom had done—and still does—for me?

My omni-patient mother kept us fed, clothed, educated, entertained, and loved way above standard. She taught us so many things beyond going potty, eating with a fork, and singing the ABCs. She taught us to love without fear; to follow our dreams; to work hard; to be compassionate; to be reliable friends; to appreciate the importance of being alive; to enjoy food, laughter, and wine; to be moved by music; to dance with abandon; to stick our bare feet in the sand and lick our salty lips; to enjoy the beautiful world we share with others—you know, the important stuff I want to teach my daughter, too. Upon reflection, when I look at my Mamafesto, I realize it was edified by my own mom's teachings. This realization brings tears to my eyes.

Sure, my mom has some faults, but it turns out her weaknesses may have made me a more independent woman and a stronger mom to my daughter. And above all, my mom's love for me is like the universe. When my mom found out Hunty had bitten my hand (I hid it from her because I wanted to go to the fair and I knew she'd make us go to the doctor instead), she took me to the hospital to get a tetanus shot. And she gets bonus points for never having been incarcerated. Take that, Martha!

Now that I've debunked Martha and "absolved" my mother, I need to work on being the most perfectly imperfect mama I can be.

Practice Makes Imperfect

Kurt Cobain once said: "Practice makes perfect, but nobody is perfect, so why practice?" Well, Kurt, because in your own words: "I'm not like them, but I can pretend." Pretending is at least trying. I just can't give myself too much of a guilt trip when I fail.

Granting ourselves permission to be (charmingly) imperfect is not the same as lowering our parenting standards. Those should always remain tall and mighty. Parents who practice ongoing neglect, carelessness, or irresponsibility; dole out any kind of abuse; or allow harm to happen to their children are to be condemned. I'd be the first to interfere if I witnessed a parent hurting or neglecting their child. Hell, I sometimes want to step in when a caregiver is talking to a child as though he's merely a genetic nuisance.

What I'm referring to is us moms learning to forgive ourselves and others. Cultivating kindness and solidarity in our parental community could perhaps eradicate some of the judgment that plagues it. Many types of judgment and guilt, both small and big, are associated with maternal insecurities. We project onto others our own supernatural expectations of what a mother should be. For example: *She didn't breastfeed/ I didn't breastfeed. She gained so much weight/I shouldn't have eaten that cheesecake. She feeds those kids too much healthy crap and the poor kid's gonna go on a binge someday/I've got to stop feeding my kid frozen chicken nuggets and fries. Her sink was just piled up with dishes/I shouldn't nap while she naps because there's so much to do around the house. She barely sees her son because she works overtime/I should really wake up an hour earlier so I can spend more time with my daughter before I go to work. She's a friggin' drone over that poor kid/I was having a good time and now I'm late to pick up my son. She spends so much money on that little girl's clothes, we could feed an entire village on her wardrobe/I spent too much on my ombré hair. She let her baby pet a stranger dog/I took my baby to a dog that almost bit her cheek off.*

Shutting out those catty voices is easier said than done and a constant conversation I have with myself. But I'm getting there. I've also gotten better at accepting myself and trusting that I'm doing the right thing. And if my good intentions backfire or I simply mess up? Well, I try to let it go and make a mental note to do better next time, to not give up.

I can't allow myself to have Cobain's "why try?" attitude—whether he was being sarcastic or not. That would be a terrible example to set for my daughter. It would be like telling her: "Oh, don't you worry about getting a good score on your SAT. Someone else will always get a better one, so why bother?"

It is in the trying that we become all we can be.

AFTERWORD:

POSTPARTUM REFLECTIONS

The Good, the Bad, and the Awesome

EVEN THOUGH we're at the end of this book, our motherhood journeys have barely begun. Before we part ways, I feel compelled to share some final tidbits I have gleaned from this crazy adventure thus far. I now understand our nurse's desire to cram in as much advice as possible before we left the hospital.

Since that momentous day, I've experienced many feelings I didn't foresee. Having had some time to process them, I've put down my reflections in hopes you find them helpful.

The Fear Parasite

Having children is not for the faint of heart. I quickly realized that I should never have taken having good nights' sleep for granted. And I'm not talking about night feedings or the many tiring physical aspects of caring for a child. What I'm alluding to is parental insomnia: the worry that comes with loving someone so much.

When my daughter was born, the term "heartbreak" took on a whole new meaning. Every time I saw her, my heart broke. And not in that sappy teenage way. I instantly developed a larger-than-life feeling for this tiny little someone who was so vulnerable to everything. Nobody warned me that becoming a parent would bring on a sudden fear of mortality.

I remember the moment it hit me. I was staring at my daughter's wrinkled newborn face, thinking she looked like a little old lady. This triggered the understanding of an inevitable truth, one so blatant I had chosen to ignore it up until that point: *If she is lucky, she will grow old and die someday. And so will I.*

"Death is the only sure thing in life," my Mamá Gloria used to say.

This haunts me. I want my daughter to live a long and happy life. And I want to *see* her live her long and happy life. The alternative is unthinkable.

I stress out over not having control of her safety on a large scale, especially facing an event like a shooting or a terrorist act. Keeping her safe in our own home is challenging enough. Some days, I irrationally fear that a knife will fall from the counter directly into her chest. So yeah, add unlikely freak accidents to the list of horrible things that can happen, and you're walking around with a beating heart carved out of your chest like in a Frida Kahlo painting.

I fight my mortality fears by concentrating on the present: holding my daughter's warm, sticky fingers in the palm of my hand, feeling her breath where her mouth intersects my neck, seeing her big belly rhythmically rise up and down as she sleeps, witnessing her excitement in inventorying the contents of each and every container in our home (over and over again), drinking in the jubilation in her voice when she whispers: "You're the best mommy I've ever seen," or recently: "I love loving you."

Experts say you should live in the present, but looking ahead also helps me. I think about the stuff greeting cards are made of: removing the training wheels from her bike, her first day of school, her first dance, maybe a wedding...and hopefully someday seeing her have a child of her own. I also like to imagine all the things I look forward to doing with her: cuddling on the couch watching movies over a bowl of parmesan-truffle popcorn, long hikes, sailing the Caribbean, yoga retreats, and of course wine-tasting trips when she's old enough. These musings help me sleep at night and keep me sane. But not for long.

The fear of failure is another force to reckon with. I'm constantly fighting worry over failing my daughter. Or doing the wrong thing and causing irreparable damage. Even stuff like putting her in PJs with flame retardants or letting her drink out of a plastic cup makes me anxious that I'm going to damage her for life. Then there's bigger stuff like: *Will giving in to her demands turn her into a brat?* My brain is filled with a loop of unanswerable questions. I try not to let these concerns take any joy out of motherhood.

I have no doubt that trying to answer these questions will be far more complicated as she gets older. So I try hard not to give in to my inner worrywart. *Don't sweat the small stuff,* I remind myself daily. *Focus on giving her a great day every day, and a happy future should follow. Deal with issues as they come, and when they do come, find the strength to let her have a hand at problem-solving.* I make myself reread my Mamafesto so as not to derail.

And while I really want my daughter to "fear no mistake" as I originally proclaimed, I'm just now starting to realize how hard it's gonna be to ride bitch while my daughter maneuvers the highway of life. Loving one's child is an unprecedented emotion. It's not the kind of love you want to set free like a bird to see if it comes back to you. It's more like having a kite you keep wanting to reel in close to you when the wind gets fierce.

The definition, boundaries, and repercussions of love are forever changed the day you hold your first child. And that's not the only mama-morphosis.

The End of an Era

When I was pregnant, people told me again and again: "Your life will be over." I didn't listen. I thought my life would remain fun and social. That I would still go out to dinner with my girlfriends and on weekly dates with my husband. That I would find time to exercise, copulate, shower, and read. And I do find time. Just not very often.

My beauty and health routines have taken a hit. Last night, I could've donated to Locks of Love all the fur I plucked out of my eyebrows. My body? I keep vowing to tone up some lingering mommy jiggles, but my frequent and intense workouts have turned into occasional "quickies." I get most of my exercise via ten-minute drills I find on the Internet (Popsugar.com/fitness is da bomb) and most of my cardio comes from pushing the stroller or carrying my daughter when she's too lazy to toddle about (which, for better or worse, happens quite often). Who needs a CrossFit vest when you have to tote a thirty-three-pound toddler?

Motherhood does provide many impromptu opportunities to burn calories. Yesterday, I had to sprint after my sitter's car for half a mile after I realized I'd left my phone on its roof (found the phone on the road, unharmed). But truth be told, I want to smack that healthy pregnant girl who started this book singing about how much exercise she got to have. Keeping an active lifestyle and minding my nutrition while I was pregnant did help me bounce back into a saggier version of my "fighting weight," but staying in line with all of that now that I'm a mom is highly impractical.

These days, I feed off my daughter's sloppy seconds—because who has the energy to be healthy all the time anymore? And making myself a salad when there's plenty of mac 'n' cheese left is just wasteful, really. (This also prevents me from eating her leftovers *in addition to* my own meal, which has happened more often than I care to admit.) At least I get in some squats during her dinner, as I usually have to pick up every other bite of hers off the floor or get up five times to cater to her highness. She's constantly wanting something "more" or the same thing "again."

And the whining. Oh, the whining. The absence of silence really hurts your ears when you become a mom. I miss quiet meals, or at least uninterrupted conversations with other adults. Dinner with girlfriends has turned into messy family buffet nights at the local Souplantation (next time I'll be bringing a flask). My beloved Bloody Mary leisure brunches on outdoor patios are now spent sprawled over a booth in an un-hip restaurant with ample parking, bad Bloody Marys, and badder coffee. (And I say stupid shit like that all the time. The other day I said: "We have two burgers to go to today.")

Because that's what your brain does when it's tired. And my brain and body and soul are all tired, all the time. Being present for my daughter can sometimes feel like a sentence; I find myself looking at the clock, counting the minutes to bedtime (a.k.a. freedom).

To spend quality time with friends, most of whom are busy riding the same baby swell, our nap schedules, errands, and family outings all need to align. When they do, it's often a lose-lose situation: If we hang out with the kids, our brains are splintered. It's hard to have a satisfying conversation while trying to keep your child from eating crayons. And if you end up having the luxury to meet without the kiddos, you hear the bomb timer ticking in the background. You're either counting the money you're spending on a sitter, or the time you'll have to make up to your partner who agreed to watch the baby. Friends without kids? Well, the love is still there, but we might as well live in different galaxies. Bedtimes, reading material, and limited spontaneity can put a dent in the best of friendships. Some of the girls I used to run with have seen my daughter fewer than three times in the three years she's been alive.

I set out wanting my life to be unchanged by motherhood, but I found out that's impossible. I didn't really know how much of myself—and my time—I would end up having to give. I'm hanging in there, though. I'm a wild salmon full of omega-3s swimming against the current. I fight every day to get time to myself. To write. To exercise. To meet with a friend. I refuse to give up hope that things will go back to my hip, pre-child life. Someday when she goes to college, I'll be able to fly by the seat of my pants again. In the meantime, I've settled for the new cool.

The New Cool

If being "cool" involves crazy raves blowing bubbles in the living room, birthday-party-hopping on weekends, and chugging wine out of red Solo cups at the park while my daughter terrorizes the fauna and flora—I've still got it.

My hip clutch rarely sees the dark of night. I can now not-so-proudly report that I don a canvas tote with a giant pocket, which is crafted in the shape of—wait for it—a kooky button-eyed owl, poised next to a decoupage flower. If you look inside the mama-bag (at your own risk), you may find a half-eaten banana, various wiping devices (some half-used), a first-aid kit, a carnage of Cherrios stuck on sticker traps, and most likely, a diaper that has collected all the hairs, boogers, and dirt that cohabit in a mom's purse. Rest assured, the diaper will inevitably land (and perish) on my daughter's butt. As far as my fashion ethics go, it's a good thing I still fit into my high school clothes, because my sense of style hasn't improved at all since then. I also still *feel* like an awkward, self-aware teenager, eager to be accepted by my peers.

When I'm with other moms, I can't help but compare myself to them. I often feel like every other mother knows something that I don't. That they've cracked the code, solved the impossible mother of all Rubik's Cubes. *How do they manage to get out of the house in a clean outfit with brushed hair and a light coat of makeup?!* I find myself marveling. *And they have three kids!* Their seeming magnificence at motherhood makes me feel like I did as the chubby outcast at volleyball camp who always got picked last. I guess I'm still a preadolescent at heart, wanting to be accepted into the cool crowd.

But if there's something I've learned by looking back at my high school years that followed, when I climbed and fell from the social ladder, it's that being cool is overrated. And oftentimes, boring—or dangerous. So my advice: Try not to give a fudge. Odds are, your kid will laugh at you no matter what. So wear your freak-flag high. Mom is the new black.

And if you hang out on the sidelines long enough, you'll find a band of misfits to populate your mom tribe. These girls will save your life.

Me, the Mom

Motherhood hits us all differently. I've become softer in some ways, both physically and emotionally. I'm more earnest and, I daresay, vulnerable. I used to see vulnerability as a sign of weakness (damn mommy issues!); now I accept it as part of being human. Admittedly, I still have a ways to go. Because let's face it: We bring all of our baggage into the motherhood motel. It's hard for me to forgive my own adult human shortcomings, let alone those of others.

The double standards are laughably hypocritical.

If my daughter's ice cream falls on the grass, I don't tell her: "Get over it—stop being a wimp!" But if my husband complains about his dish not having enough butter...well, let's just say I don't hug him tight and say, "I'm so sorry. Mama will get you another one." It's hard to remember those mom skills out in the world. But when I do, they make me a more compassionate friend, spouse, stranger.

I try to exercise compassion towards myself, too. I can't be calling myself stupid. I wouldn't want my daughter to follow in those self-deprecating footsteps that lead to low self-esteem. And this is very hard, because for someone who used to pride herself on being "on top of it," I make so many mistakes that I unfortunately can't blame on my "mommy brain" (a term that irks me because I think mom's brains are awesome). Yeah, my noodle isn't functioning at full capacity (whether from growing a human or lack of sleep), but my mom fails are a whole new beast of personal shortcomings I find difficult to overcome.

For example, Ms. Nutrition (yours truly) just got schooled by the pediatrician on Toddler Feeding 101. Apparently, I've been giving my daughter ten times the (organic) starches she should consume. "It's not the quality of the nutrition but the quantity that's a problem," she told me on the last visit. So yeah, I get to eat crow now, too. And maybe I *did* turn my daughter into an emotional eater by breastfeeding her on demand. But I'm getting better at focusing my energy on improving rather than allowing myself to drown in guilt quicksand.

I still strive to be a cut above my own folks, and as a result, I hope I'm becoming a more considerate daughter—one who is more understanding, more forgiving, and way less judgmental. I now understand why my mom accidentally set fire to the kitchen two times (I almost burned mine down today) and never bothered to do our hair. Judging by my little one who doesn't slow down for the brush, I can't imagine running after three such creatures. Mine is often the only girl in a room without some sort of hair arrangement. I ask myself: *Who the F—err—hel-heck cares?* (Really trying to curb that cussing.) But I do care! I fear being judged by all the other moms in ballet class. It's hard to overcome that worry of not belonging.

Mom politics and parenting philosophies are insane! Helicopter, free-range, attachment, RIE, slow, permissive...who can keep up? Have we become too precious about parenting? I'm just grateful if I make it through the day with a happy, healthy girl tucked safely in bed!

I've learned to trust my instincts over whatever new thinking is hip. *If* I have the time, I read about it to at least feel in-the-know and borrow what feels right to me. I totally want to excel at this thing, but how people survived without parenting coaches and sleep trainers in the past is mind-boggling. Totally being sarcastic here— though I've been tempted to bring in someone to help me get my daughter to sleep in past four-thirty in the morning.

Motherhood has made me honest, too. Annoyingly so. The other day, I received two Learning Towers by mistake. I was tempted to profit from the oversight; I'm fairly certain that, once upon a time, I would've sold that highly coveted merch on Craigslist. Instead,

I returned it to its rightful owner. I can't teach honesty while contrabanding.

Very much a survival instinct, motherhood turns us into the mom we need to be at a particular moment: noble, strong, funny, thoughtful, sober, responsible, or even a badass, should the need arise.

Me, the Human Being

Being good at this mom thing doesn't mean I get to forget myself along the way. I can't be the best mom possible if I'm not fulfilled. For me, being happy includes being known as something other than a mom. I want to be an individual, first and foremost. I want to remain the girl my husband fell in love with. I want to be the kind of lady my daughter could aspire to be someday. Most importantly, I want to die as the old woman I wanted to grow up to be.

I'm making my own "mom mold" as I go along, shaped in its own unique way that fits me. And I try not to care what other moms think of it or what their molds look like. I have my own needs, dreams, and passions. And I can't—won't—allow any kind of guilt to arise from pursuing any of those things. I like to watch movies, I enjoy taking pictures and going on hikes, I need massages from time to time, I love to write, and to teach, and I hope to direct a feature film someday. I try to put as much time into pursuing these goals as I do into fulfilling my daughter's needs. This is very hard, because I need and want to give so much of my soul to her (not to mention that hanging out with my daughter is often easier than doing a rewrite). But if I give it *all* to her, then at some point, I'll have emptied myself beyond recognition. Plus, she deserves a happy mom. A mom focused on the big life picture versus what kind of sleep training one should be employing. (But in case you're wondering, when our daughter was about five months old, we did a combination of "cry it out" and "The Happy Sleeper" [per the book by Heather Turgeon and Julie Wright]. Our daughter was sleeping through the night in two days.)

My mom-job requirements don't include stashing my hopes and dreams and hard-earned education into the basement with my cheesy Catholic girl Halloween costume. I've become a good juggler of parental, romantic, and professional responsibilities. When I get overwhelmed by one function, I move on to the next function. That's how all the balls are kept in motion. And, yeah, when I drop one, I throw it back into the air with my feet. I always try to leave a little room for self-care, too. And when self-doubt comes around the corner, I open a bottle of wine to drown my self-pity in and talk to my friends about self-improvement. I wake up with purpose and a hangover.

Being a woman, a mom, or a spouse doesn't have to be the only thing that defines me as an individual. Of course each of them is an intricate part of the person I am today, but if you were to strip away all of those, surely something would be left of me. At least I'd like to think so.

Me, the Wife

My husband and I have known each other for fifteen years. In those years we've been friends, confidants, lovers, estranged, lovers again, married, and currently, parents to the most amazing little girl I always knew I wanted. But when we built our relationship, we didn't cement it on a baby or even the possibility of a baby.

Having a child doesn't necessarily make a relationship better or worse, stronger or weaker. It simply adds texture to it. Sometimes this texture is so fulfilling, you can't imagine life in any other form. Being a family together on top of being a couple is magnificent. Group hugs stop being sitcom-worthy saccharine displays of affections, farts are uproariously celebrated, and the third wheel makes the ol' bike a shiny new trike.

However, other times this texture feels like camping out in the cold rain in a sleeping bag made of sandpaper. Sloppy kisses get you sick, bowel movements are no longer private, and that third wheel makes you forget how smooth it was to ride without the extra cargo.

It's hard to be your best self for your partner when you spend a lot of your good stuff on your child. Some people say you must put your significant other first, before your child, and I don't entirely disagree. But I sometimes fail in favor of our daughter. I keep trying to balance the scale, because I know how important it is to be a good partner. This lesson was engrained in me during my parents' divorce when my father confided in me that my mom was always a great mother but not always a good wife. Of course, to him this meant that a five-course meal wasn't ready when he walked through the door or that she welcomed him in ratty, unflattering pajamas (standards by which my relationship would also be broken). But the fact is that my father felt that his needs (however ridiculous and chauvinistic) weren't being met, and that is a takeaway worth remembering.

My parents grew apart because they failed to grow *together*. They tried to talk, but they didn't listen to each other. They let stubbornness stand in the way of self-improvement. I don't want that to happen to me. If my husband says to me: "I like your hair better in a ponytail than in a bun." I make the effort to remember this when I'm pulling back my hair. If he asks me not to leave my floss lying around because it's gross, I try to remember to throw it in the trash. And I constantly try (and fail) not to leave the sink faucet on hot. Making little adjustments can go a long way; otherwise, they may add up to something hard to overcome. Hopefully, my losing my phone every week won't be a deal-breaker because that's just something I don't think I'll ever "quit."

The quality of my "wifehood" falters from time to time, and I have to tack consistently so my sails don't lose wind. I struggle to stay current, interesting (and interested), fit, hairless in the right places, sexually available, and just plain friendly. Most of these things don't come innately to me, so I have to push myself to read that hot article, or to enjoy his baseball game CliffsNotes, or to shave my legs, or to avoid adding things to my shopping list while having sex, or simply to remember that this is the man I chose to spend my life with. He is smart, sexy, funny (though I'm funnier for sure), talented, considerate, loyal, interesting, and a sensational dad. Plus, he plays the guitar.

My love for the father of my child is the reason she is here, enhancing our experience in this earth. I try to keep my sights on that. I also want our daughter to have a healthy example of what a romantic relationship is supposed to be.

Amorous relationships are born out of attraction, common interests, compatibility, and respect. They grow with patience, trust, care, communication, and intimacy. Maintaining a good relationship takes effort. Being a good partner is something to take pride in. I want my daughter to learn all of these things and to have the opportunity to experience healthy romantic love in her own life, regardless of what number she puts in the "dependents" box of her tax form. Which means, she can't always be part of the equation when it comes to my relationship, even when we all belong to the same family.

Oh, Shit (and Other Joys of Motherhood)

When I turned in my initial draft of this book to my first editor, it was returned with one big general question: "What are the joys of motherhood?"

I laughed. I shared the comment with other moms. They laughed, too. I guess you have to be a mom to implicitly know that for every single tear of despair and frustration you'll shed, you'll imbibe a magnum bottle of effervescent, soul-altering, intoxicating joy.

Motherhood is hard, sometimes downright ugly. As bestselling author Naomi Wolf summed up in *Misconceptions: Truth, Lies, and the Unexpected on the Journey to Motherhood*: "Giving birth is natural—but becoming a mother in its deepest sense is *not* exclusively natural." Whereas I didn't struggle with postpartum depression like Naomi, I *have* found motherhood to be trying. It is a challenging life adjustment, no matter how much you plan, want, and love your baby.

As well-stated by Maria Guido on the Scary Mommy website: "If we'd all stop pretending growing a human and caring for it 24/7 was so enjoyable and easy, we'd be better off."

So with that in mind, while writing this book, I focused on a lot of the trying aspects of motherhood, because I wanted to depict a realistic picture for those of us who didn't realize how hard it would really be. I also wanted to share my ups and downs and motivate others to find their own way through the glitterless mother-maze without fear of judgment. I wanted to create a safe space where moms can "be." I had made the assumption that all the perks that came with motherhood were obvious. But just in case...

MOTHERHOOD: THE ADVENTURE OF A LIFETIME

"Oh, shit," my daughter said in church. She was with her grandparents who never skip Sunday Mass. I was sad to miss it (the "Oh, shit," not the Mass), but I could clearly envision her pot-bellied self, happily toddling about, clutching the strap of her backpack with her dimpled little hands as she dragged it down the aisle. Until it caught on a pew. The mishap caused her to mutter the expletive that will be a beloved family story for generations to come. My favorite part was that she didn't phrase it with an exclamation point. Deadpan. And inappropriately profane, just like her mama during Parent and Me music class when I realized the parking meter had been left unfed. What more could a mother ask for, right? (Besides a lifetime supply of patience, massage gift certificates, dark chocolate, and red wine.)

Motherhood is the most amazing thing that's ever happened to me. I love being a mother. I even came to love breastfeeding so much that I nursed my daughter 'til she was almost two years old. I loved spending every morning with her face nuzzled in my arms as she fed, her chubby little fingers pumping my shriveled boobs. I lived for the occasional look-and-smile between gulps. This is from the woman who swore to never nurse past the day when baby could say "boobie." Guess who totally gulped those words. *Ahem.*

My daughter has also rekindled my imagination in ways only a child can. She has taught me that an ordinary leaf can be an extraordinary vessel for rocks or that a bath toy can double as a yummy taco. This is some *Matrix* shit.

Because of her, I see the world differently. And it scares me more than it used to. But at the same time, I want to make it a better place. For her. And unbeknownst to her, she helps me do this.

Her bravery and determination keep me on my toes and inspire me to push harder in my own life. I'm amazed at her ability to pick herself up after a fall. And at the tenacity and strength she exerts to scale gym walls, furniture, and steep flights of stairs. When I see her huffing and puffing, determined to get to the top, I remember those gruesome P.E. classes where our teacher made us climb the school bleachers over and over again. I can't tell you how many times I just gave up. But she, she just keeps going. She's unstoppable, and the trust she bestows upon me is humbling.

It's difficult not being able to express yourself and having to rely on others to feed you, bathe you, nurse you, understand you, entertain you, and move you from place to place. I mean, I would hate to have to depend on someone else to fulfill my basic needs. Yet, she patiently allows me to do the best I can to keep her happy, healthy, and safe.

The girl's a riot, too. She makes me laugh harder than my pelvic floor can handle. Her laughter is the soundtrack I hope to hear on my way to heaven. Then, I'll know I got in.

Being a mom is fun. Especially if you're a bit egocentric like me. No one has ever been so engaged by my singing and dancing abilities (or lack thereof) as my daughter. She's my number one fan. And I'm hers. Well, I guess she's got two number one fans because her daddy is madly in love with her, too. I love seeing those two together.

On a normal day, Dad picks her up from daycare while I get dinner ready. I peek constantly out the window, waiting for that car to pull up. I get giddy. I know she's looking forward to this moment like she anticipates a good tickle session. When they pull up, I open the door and wave enthusiastically at her. She's already smiling, but when she sees me, her smile stretches out. "I've never seen her smile that way except when she looks at you," my husband told me the other night. Her toothy grin kills me and then brings me back to life, renewed. She's the most wonderful thing in the world. Every parent thinks their kid is the bee's knees; well, my daughter is the *whole* bee, its hive, and all the pollen on earth.

Every time my daughter runs to me with her arms outstretched, I remember dreams of catching this very child, from before I was her mom. Every night as I tuck her in, I tell her that I always wanted a little girl *just* like her. I couldn't possibly love her more. Except that every new day, I do. I'd heard about unconditional love ad nauseam, but it wasn't until the day I pushed her into this world that I understood all the implications of the cliché. I'll keep pushing for her 'til I die. I love her immensely and infinitely. No. Matter. What.

I already owe her so much. I didn't know I was able to be so unselfish. I didn't know I could be so patient. She's made me a better being. She's helped me overcome my fear of dogs. If it weren't for her, I would never have had the courage to take some calculated risks of my own. She inspired me to quit a job that made me miserable. Motherhood made me brave enough to face myself in order to write this book. I had to dig deep and expose my vulnerability, which has left me publicly naked in a dressing room with unforgiving mirrors and lights. But now, I can see past the reflection and cellulite into the person inside the shell. It's me. It's always been me. It's just that now I'm a mom, too.

And it's all so bittersweet: My little girl is not all mine. She belongs to me, to her dad, to the world, and to her own bright and beautiful self.

They tell you that it all goes by so quickly. Every day, I savor her every breath, her every thought, her every milestone. I'm already nostalgic for yesterday. But I'm also looking forward to tomorrow. Having a child is that powerful. I hold the past, present, and future when I hug my daughter.

Her name is Phaedra.

BIBLIOGRAPHY

CHAPTER 1: MY EJACULATE CONCEPTION

Anderson, B. L., E. P. Dang, R. L. Floyd, R. Sokol, J. Mahoney, and J. Schulkin. "Knowledge, Opinions, and Practice Patterns of Obstetrician-gynecologists regarding Their Patients' Use of Alcohol." *Journal of Addiction Medicine* (U.S. National Library of Medicine), June 4, 2010.

Black, Ronald A., M.D., and D. Ashley Hill, M.D. "Over-the-Counter Medications in Pregnancy." *Over-the-Counter Medications in Pregnancy – American Family Physician*, June 15, 2003.

Bowen, Michael. "Chromosome Abnormalities in Pregnancy." *Netdoctor* (Hearst Magazines U.K.), November 10, 2015.

Cohen-Overbeek, T.E., M.D., M. Den Ouden, M.D., L. Pijpers, M.D., M.G. J. Jahoda, M.D., J.W. Waldimiroff, M.D., and W.C.J. Hop, MSC. "Spontaneous Abortion Rate and Advanced Maternal Age: Consequences for Prenatal Diagnosis." *Science Direct*, July 7, 1990. Originally published in *The Lancet*. 336.876 (1990): 27–29.

Corbett, Holly C. "Safe Medications to Take While Pregnant." *Fit Pregnancy and Baby*, April 3, 2017.

Crandall, B. F., and C. Chua. "Detecting Neural Tube Defects by Amniocentesis between 11 and 15 Weeks' Gestation." *Prenatal Diagnosis* (U.S. National Library of Medicine), April 14, 1995.

de la Cretaz, Britni. "Common Chromosomal Abnormalities That Can Cause Miscarriage." *Romper,* May 4, 2016.

Danielsson, Krissi. "Can Low-Dose Aspirin Prevent Miscarriages?" *Verywell,* May 6, 2016.

Danielsson, Krissi. "Can Progesterone Administration Prevent Miscarriages?" *Verywell,* January 31, 2017.

Danielsson, Krissi. "What Do Miscarriage Statistics Really Mean?" *Verywell,* April 28, 2016.

Danielsson, Krissi. "Why Do Chromosomal Abnormalities Cause Miscarriage?" *Verywell,* January 31, 2017.

Dashiell, Andrea. "Miscarriage: Causes, Signs, and What to Expect." *Parents,* July 29, 2015.

"18–20 Week Pregnancy Ultrasound." *BabyCenter.* September 2014.

Ghidini, Alessandro, M.D. "Patient Education: Chorionic Villus Sampling (Beyond the Basics)." *Up To Date,* April 16, 2015.

Keller, Nathan A., and Asha Rijshinghani. "Advantages of the Quadruple Screen over Noninvasive Prenatal Testing." *Clinical Case Reports,* March, 2016.

Kiefer, Amy. "Lies, Damned Lies, and Miscarriage Statistics." *Expecting Science,* March 11, 2016.

Koren, G., S. Madjunkova, and C. Maltepe. "The Protective Effects of Nausea and Vomiting of Pregnancy against Adverse Fetal Outcome— a Systematic Review." *National Center for Biotechnology Information* (U.S. National Library of Medicine), August 2014.

Ljunger, E., S. Cnattingius, C. Lundin, and G. Annerén. "Chromosomal Anomalies in First-trimester Miscarriages." *National Center for Biotechnology Information* (U.S. National Library of Medicine), November 2005.

Makrydimas, G., N. J. Sebire, D. Lolis, N. Vlassis, and K. H. Nicolaides. "Fetal Loss Following Ultrasound Diagnosis of a Live Fetus at 6–10 Weeks of Gestation." *Ultrasound in Obstetrics & Gynecology,* September 2, 2003.

"Miscarriage: Signs, Symptoms, Treatment and Prevention." *American Pregnancy Association,* August 30, 2016.

Oster, Emily. "I Wrote That It's OK to Drink While Pregnant. Everyone Freaked Out. Here's Why I'm Right." *Slate Magazine,* September 11, 2013.

Relevant, Julie. "Itchy Skin during Pregnancy Should Not Be Ignored." *Fox News*, April 13, 2017.

"Rh Factor." *American Pregnancy Association,* March 2, 2017.

Stone, Joanne, M.D. "SMFM Consult: Risks of Chorionic Villus Sampling and Amniocentesis." *Contemporary OB/GYN*, February 1, 2014.

"Sudafed during Pregnancy." *PregMed*, November 26, 2014.

Thompson, Trisha. "Seven Most Common Miscarriage Causes." *Parents,* August 16, 2016.

Walton, Alice G. "Morning Sickness May Be Linked To A Healthier Pregnancy." *Forbes,* September 27, 2016.

"Why Miscarriages Happen – Often We Never Know Why." *Miscarriage Support Auckland NZ*, n.d.

CHAPTER 3: PRENATAL HEALTH &
CHAPTER 4: BRING IT ON, JANE FONDA

Antonow-Schlorkea, Iwa, Matthias Schwaba, Laura Coxb, Kristina Stuchlika, Otto W. Wittea, Peter W. Nathanielszc, and Thomas J. McDonald. "Vulnerability of the Fetal Primate Brain to Moderate Reduction in Maternal Global Nutrient Availability." *PNAS,* December 21, 2010.

Asprey, Lana, M.D., and Dave Asprey. *The Better Baby Book: How to Have a Healthier, Smarter, Happier Baby.* John Wiley & Sons, Inc. 2013.

Bouchez, Colette. "Exercise During Pregnancy: Myth vs. Fact." *WebMD,* February 6, 2009.

"Calcium for Pregnancy: Diet & Supplements." *Cleveland Clinic,* February 11, 2016.

"Calcium in Your Pregnancy Diet." *Baby Center,* 2015.

"Calcium Supplementation in Pregnant Women." *World Health Organization,* 2013.

Castro, Giselle. "5 Healthy Grains With More Protein Than Quinoa." *Women's Health Mag,* August 20, 2014.

"Choose the Right Fish To Lower Mercury Risk Exposure." *Consumer Reports,* August 2014.

DeNoon, Daniel J. "The Truth About Vitamin D: What Kind of Vitamin D is Best?" *WebMD,* n.d.

"Energy and Protein Intake in Pregnancy." *World Health Organization,* October 31, 2003.

"Five Foods that Contain Monosaturated Fat." *Fit Day,* n.d.

"Folate Dosing." *Mayo Clinic,* February 1, 2014.

Fox, Isadora. "The Benefits of Walking for Pregnant and New Moms." *Parents*, n.d. Originally published in *American Baby Magazine,* August 2004.

"Guideline: Calcium supplementation in pregnant women." *World Health Organization,* 2013.

Haiken, Melanie, M.A. "Iron and Pregnancy." *Health Day,* March 11, 2015.

"Healthy Diet During Pregnancy." *Healthline,* March 29, 2016.

Juhasz, Francine. "The Effects of Poor Nutrition on a Fetus." *Livestrong,* August 16, 2013.

Kashtan, Paula. "Q&A: Calcium During Pregnancy" *The Bump,* 2015.

Kelly, D., T. O'Dowd, and U. Reulbash. "Use of folic acid supplements and risk of cleft lip and palate in infants: a population-based cohort study." National Center for Biotechnology Information (U.S. National Library of Medicine), July 2012.

Kiefer, David. "Whey Protein." *WebMD*, May 1, 2015.

Kresser, Chris, M.S., L.Ac. "5 Myths About Pregnancy Nutrition." *Healthy Baby Code,* 2011.

"Information on the Latest Vitamin D News and Research." *Vitamin D Council*, January 30, 2013.

"Iron." *U.S. National Library of Medicine*, n.d.

Levine, J.A. "Non-exercise Activity Thermogenesis (NEAT)." *National Center for Biotechnology Information* (U.S. National Library of Medicine), December 16, 2002.

Luscombe, Belinda. "True or False? 20 Common Myths about Pregnancy." *Time,* May 5, 2011.

Lynch, Amy. "5 Benefits of Prenatal Yoga." *Mind Body Green,* May 4, 2012.

"Magnesium." *Office of Dietary Supplements – National Institutes of Health*, February 11, 2016.

Mattheis, Christine. "14 Non-Dairy Foods That Are High in Calcium." *Health*, n.d.

"MCT Oil: What You Need To Know." *Paleo Leap*, n.d.

Morrison, Amy. "20 Things They Don't Tell You About Your Pregnant Body." *Scary Mommy*, January 22, 2015.

Myers, Wyatt. "NEAT Exercises for Couch Potatoes." *Everyday Health*, November 7, 2012.

Narins, Elizabeth. "Sunscreen Doesn't Stop Vitamin D Production." *Women's Health*, June 20, 2013.

"Nutrition, Carbohydrate and Calorie Counter." *CalorieKing*, n.d.

"Omega-3 Fatty Acids." *University of Maryland Medical Center*, August 5, 2015.

"Omega-3 Fish Oil and Pregnancy: Benefits & Proper Dosage." *American Pregnancy Association*, July 2015.

Pevzner, Holly. "7 Crazy Things That Happen to Your Vagina During Pregnancy." *Parents*, n.d.

"Pilates in Pregnancy." *Baby Center*, n.d.

Pratt, Steven. *SuperfoodsRX for Pregnancy: The Right Choices for a Healthy, Smart, Super Baby.* New Jersey: John Wiley & Sons, 2013.

"Prenatal Vitamin Limits & Recommendations." *American Pregnancy Association*, April 26, 2012.

"Prenatal yoga: What you need to know." *Mayo Clinic*, January 22, 2015.

Raffelock, Dean, M.D. "The Truth About Vitamin A Safety in Prenatal Vitamins." *Care2 Healthy Living*, August 22, 2010.

Sass, Cynthia, RD. "Best Shape: Eat Slim at Every Age." *Health Magazine*, April 2, 2016.

Snyder, Kimberly. "The 7 Nutrients You Need While Pregnant (and Which Foods to Avoid)." *Kimberly Snyder*, n.d.

"Vitamin D and Pregnancy: What Are the Benefits?" *American Pregnancy Association*, April 24, 2013.

"Vitamin D in your pregnancy diet." *Baby Center*, 2015.

"Weight Gain Concerns During Pregnancy." *American Pregnancy Association*, April 26, 2012.

"Why is protein important during pregnancy?" *Mommi*, n.d.

Witty, Tracey, ed. "B12 and Pregnancy." *B12 Deficiency*, n.d.

Ziel, Erica. "Can I lie on my back while pregnant?" *Knocked-Up Fitness*, April 18, 2013.

CHAPTER 5: SEX, LIES, AND MASTURBATE

Brown, Melissa. "18 Best Sex Positions While Pregnant." *Cafe Mom*, July 24, 2012.

Daubney, Martin. "A Husband Confesses: 'Seeing My Wife Give Birth Put Me off Sex for a YEAR!'" *Daily Mail Online*, November 1, 2012.

Delvin, David. "Anal Sex." *Netdoctor* (Hearst Magazines U.K.), November 25, 2013.

Outside Providence. Miramax, 1999.

"Pregnancy Week by Week – Sex During Pregnancy." *Mayo Clinic*, July 31, 2015.

Winder, Kelly. "Libido and Breastfeeding – Where did my sex drive go?" *BellyBelly*, October 26, 2015.

CHAPTER 6: MY GREEN ALTER-MAMA

Achenbach, Joel. "107 Nobel Laureates Sign Letter Blasting Greenpeace over GMOs." *Washington Post*, June 30, 2016.

Adams, Jill U. "Are Parabens and Phthalates Harmful in Makeup and Lotions?" *Washington Post*, September 1, 2014.

"Are Flame Retardants Toxic?" *DrWeil.com*, October 9, 2014.

Bhandari, Smitha, ed. "Food Dye and ADHD: Food Coloring, Sugar, and Diet." *WebMD*, November 18, 2014.

Brown, Elizabeth. "Why Natural Deodorant Makes You Smell Like Butt." *Tonic*, 2017.

Bushart, Sean, Ph.D. "PCBs in the Air: What Are the Risks?" *Clearwater*, January 1, 1997.

Children's Health Team, ed. "Health Essentials: Can Wearing Fire-Retardant Pajamas Affect Your Child's Health?" *Health Cleveland Clinic*, December 2, 2014.

"Colors to Die For: The Dangerous Impact of Food Coloring." *Special Education Degree Net*, n.d.

"Diaper Facts." *Real Diaper Association*, May 14, 2015.

"Dioxins." *Tox Town* (U.S. National Library of Medicine), n.d.

Dwivedi, Kshama, and Girjesh Kumar. "Genetic Damage Induced by a Food Coloring Dye (Sunset Yellow) on Meristematic Cells of Brassica Campestris L." *Journal of Environmental and Public Health*, April 14, 2015.

"F.D.A. Limits Red Dye No. 3." *The New York Times*, January 29, 1990.

Freedhoff, Yoni. "The Incredible Arrogance of Thinking 'Natural' Means 'Good.'" *U.S. News*, August 21, 2013.

"GMO Education." *Responsible Technology*, n.d.

Graves, Ginny. "A Smart Guide to Scary Chemicals," *Health Magazine*, December 2015.

Greaves, Jeff. "Dangers of Coloring Hair While Pregnant." *HealthNewsDigest.com*, December 10, 2009.

"Guide to Maternal & Child Health." *Pittsburgh: Women for a Healthy Environment Organization*, n.d.

"Impact of Fluoride on Neurological Development in Children." *Harvard School of Public Health*, July 25, 2012.

Keefer, Amber. "Environmental Impact of Disposable Diapers." *Livestrong*, June 24, 2015.

Kollipara, Puneet. "Proof He's the Science Guy: Bill Nye Is Changing His Mind about GMOs." *Washington Post*, March 3, 2015.

"Laureates Letter Supporting Precision Agriculture (GMOs)." *Support Precision Agriculture*, June 29, 2016.

Lee, Jolie. "What You Need to Know about GMOs." *USA Today*, January 3, 2014.

Manitsas, Andrea. "5 Reasons We Heart Glass Over Plastic." *Organic Authority*, November 23, 2011.

"Perfluorinated Compounds (PFCs)." *WA Toxics*, n.d.

"Polychlorinated Biphenyls (PCBs)." *Illinois Department of Public Health*, 2009.

"Polychlorinated Biphenyls (PCBs) and Your Health." *Wisconsin Department of Health Services*, August 11, 2014.

Potera, Carol. "DIET AND NUTRITION: The Artificial Food Dye Blues." *Environmental Health Perspectives,* October 2010.

Pratt, Steven. *SuperfoodsRx for Pregnancy: The Right Choices for a Healthy Smart, Super Baby.* New Jersey: John Wiley & Sons, 2013.

Richardson, Jill. "Toxins in Huggies and Pampers Aren't What You Want to Put Near Baby's Skin." *Alternet*, February 18, 2014.

"SAP. (a sticky subject?)" *GDiapers Blog*, October 7, 2011.

"Seeing Red: Report Finds FDA Fails to Protect Children in Light of New Evidence on Food Dyes." *CSPI Net*, January 19, 2016.

Shames, Richard L., M.D., and Karilee H. Shames, Ph.D., RN. "We Changed Our Minds About Fluoridation: Here's Why." *Verywell*, December 4, 2014.

"6 Reasons to Use Green Cleaning Products for Your Home." *AbesMarket*, March 13, 2013.

"36 Foods That Help Detox and Cleanse Your Entire Body." *EatLocalGrown*, n.d.

Toxins in Utero Chart. *Environmental Defense Fund,* 2012.

Plus1Please. *Types of Cloth Diapers.* Posted on YouTube, n.d.

"Volatile Organic Compounds (VOCs) – Toxic Chemicals and Environmental Health Risks Where You Live and Work." *Tox Town* (U.S. National Library of Medicine), December 16, 2015.

Waits, Kentin. "6 Reasons Why Used Is Better." *Wise Bread*, September 23, 2011.

"Why Buy Locally Owned?" *Sustainable Connections*, n.d.

Young, Sandra, OD. "GMO and the Nutritional Content of Food." *Discovery Eye Foundation*, March 24, 2016.

CHAPTER 7: SERIOUSLY.

"Baby Registry Checklist." *Baby Center*, n.d.

Deardorff, Julie. "Why Physical Therapists Hate the Bumbo Baby Seat." *Chicago Tribune*, March 15, 2012.

"Must-Have Baby Registry Checklist." *Babies R Us*, n.d.

Velez, Mandy. "21 Oft-Overlooked, Must-Have Items For Your Baby Registry." *The Huffington Post*, October 8, 2014.

"What NOT to Put on a Baby Registry?" *Baby Center*, November 11, 2013.

CHAPTER 8: LABOR A LA CARTA & CHAPTER 9: WE MAKE PLANS AND GOD LAUGHS AT OUR VAGINAS

"About Meconium Aspiration." *Kids Health,* October 2014.

Andrews, Michelle. "States Vary On What They Allow Midwives To Do." *NPR*, February 14, 2012.

Ashton, Jennifer, M.D. "Study Raises Concern That Pitocin May Harm Babies." *ABC News*, May 10, 2013.

Basu, Maya, Dot Smith, and Robin Edwards. "Can the Incidence of Obstetric Anal Sphincter Injury Be Reduced? The STOMP Experience." *European Journal of Obstetrics & Gynecology and Reproductive Technology,* July 2016.

"Be the Match." *National Marrow Donor Program,* n.d.

Ben-Joseph, Elana Pearl, ed. "Circumcision." *KidsHealth*, March 2013.

Block, Jennifer. *Pushed: The Painful Truth about Childbirth and Modern Maternity Care.* Cambridge, MA: Da Capo Lifelong, 2007.

"Breech Babies: What Can I Do If My Baby Is Breech?" *Family Doctor*, November 2015.

Buckley, Sarah. "Epidurals: Risks and Concerns for Mother and Baby." *Sarah Buckley*, July 28, 2016.

Buffardi, Danielle. "The Benefits of a Vaginal Delivery." *Pregnancy Blog American Pregnancy Association,* February 3, 2012.

Buser, Genevieve L., MDCM, Sayonara Mató, MD, Alexia Y. Zhang, MPH, Ben J. Metcalf, Ph.D., Bernard Beall, Ph.D., and Ann R. Thomas, MD. "Morbidity and Mortality Weekly Report (MMWR)." *Centers for Disease Control and Prevention,* June 29, 2017.

Butler, Kiera. "Did Having a Baby Leave You with a Horrible, Debilitating, Embarrassing Injury? You're Not Alone." *Mother Jones*, February 2017.

"Cesarean Procedure: Risks & Complications for Mother & Baby." *American Pregnancy*, April 25, 2012.

Dekker, Rebecca. "Is Erythromycin Eye Ointment Always Necessary for Newborns?" *Evidence Based Birth*, November 11, 2012.

Dennehy, Kathleen. "What To Expect When You Aren't Expecting." *The Huffington Post,* January 4, 2017.

"Effacement, Dilation and Station." *Babies Online*, n.d.

"8 Registry Items You Might Forget." *Mom 365*, n.d.

"Epidural Anesthesia." *American Pregnancy Association*, August 2015.

Gaskin, Ina May. "Induced and Seduced: The Dangers of Cytotec." *Mothering*, July/August 2001.

Gatewood, Johanzynn. "Wait to Cut Umbilical Cord, Experts Urge." *CNN*, March 3, 2017.

Goodman, Brenda. "Data Shines a Light on C-sections, Maternal Mortality." *Health Journalism*, May 13, 2014.

Grant, Kelli B. "Is Cord Blood Banking Worth The Cost? Here's What the Experts Say." *NBC News*, July 29, 2015.

Haelle, Tara. "Here's The Truth About Vitamin K For Newborns." *Forbes,* August 22, 2016.

Hirsch, Larissa, M.D. "About the Apgar Score." *Kids Health*, July 2014.

"How Common Is PTSD?" *U.S. Department of Veteran Affairs,* n.d.

"How Many Women Really Get PPD?" *Postpartum Progress*, n.d.

"Is Erythromycin Eye Ointment Always Necessary for Newborns?" *Evidence Based Birth*, n.d.

Jackson, Kama Lee. "Women in Labor Stop Pushing, See Amazing Results." *Mothering*, May 8, 2017.

Jaslow, Ryan. "Not Cutting Umbilical Cord Immediately May Boost Baby's Health." *CBSNews*, July 11, 2013.

"Kids. Cutting the Cord." *Parents,* December 2015.

Koklu, Esad, Tuncay Tascale, Selmin Koklu, and Erdal Avni Ariguloglu. "Anaphylactic Shock Due to Vitamin K in a Newborn and Review of Literature." Taylor & Francis, October 17, 2013. *The Journal of Maternal-Fetal & Neonatal Medicine* 27.11 (2014): n.p.

Kopelman, Arthur E., M.D. "Meconium Aspiration Syndrome." *Merck Manuals*, n.d.

Kresser, Chris, M.S., L.Ac. "Natural Childbirth vs. Epidural Side Effects and Risks." *Chris Kresser*, August 5, 2011.

"Labor & Delivery: Types of Episiotomy." *Healthline.* Kelbach, Janine, RNC-OB, reviewer, January 28, 2016.

Lee, Bruce Y. "CDC Case Report: If You Eat Your Placenta, This Can Happen." *Forbes,* June 30, 2017.

Leeder, Jessica. "Post-traumatic (childbirth) stress disorder." *Todays Parent*, July 27, 2015.

"Let's Talk About: Circumcision and Penis Care." *Intermountain Healthcare, Primary Children's Medical Center,* 2013.

Lieberman, Ellice, and Carol O'Donoghue. "Unintended Effects of Epidural Analgesia during Labor: A Systematic Review." *American Journal of Obstetrics and Gynecology* 186.5 (2002): n.p.

Lippi, Giuseppe, and Massimo Franchini. "Vitamin K in Neonates: Facts and Myths." *Blood Transfusion,* January 2011.

Martinko, Katherine. "'Lotus Birth' Advocates Leave the Umbilical Cord Attached to Newborn Babies." *TreeHugger*, February 18, 2015.

McAuley, David. "Oxytocin (Pitocin ®)." *Global RPh,* April 4, 2015.

"Narcotics for Pain During Labor: Types & Side Effects." *American Pregnancy Association,* April 26, 2012.

Nierenberg, Cari. "Is the Baby Coming? 6 Signs of Labor." *Live Science*, January 21, 2015.

Nierenberg, Cari. "Vaginal Birth vs. C-Section: Pros & Cons." *Live Science*, March 20, 2015.

O'Connell, Meaghan. "18 Women on What Contractions Really Feel Like." *NY Mag The Cut*, March 26, 2015.

Ogbru, Omudhome, PharmD. "Oxytocin, Pitocin." *Medicine Net*, March 19, 2015.

Online Etymology Dictionary, n.d.

Pearson, Catherine. "Pitocin Risks? Study Raises Concern About Drug's Safety During Childbirth." *The Huffington Post*, July 5, 2013.

Perlstein, David, M.D. "What Is Newborn Circumcision? Circumcision: Learn the Pros and Cons of This Procedure." *MedicineNet*, November 6, 2016.

Plevin, Rebecca. "PriceCheck: Is It Cost-effective to Use a Birthing Center?" *Southern California Public Radio*, July 22, 2015.

Pope, Sarah. "Skip That Newborn Vitamin K Shot." *The Healthy Home Economist,* March 27, 2017.

"PROPYLENE GLYCOL." *EWG.* Environmental Working Group, n.d.

The Rolling Stones. "You Can't Always Get What You Want," by Mick Jagger and Keith Richards. *Let It Bleed.* Decca Records, 1969.

"Say No to Circumcision." *Circumcision Decision,* n.d.

Shanley, Laura Kaplan. "Don't Push the River, It Flows by Itself." *Unassisted Childbirth*, n.d.

"The Signs and Stages of Labor." *ARK-LA-TEX UROLOGY*, 2017.

"The Truth About Walking Epidurals." *Parenting,* n.d.

Tuteur, Amy, M.D. "The Myths of Natural Childbirth." *Time*, October 12, 2011.

"Using Epidural Anesthesia During Labor: Benefits and Risks." *American Pregnancy Association*, August 30, 2016.

"Vaginal Misoprostol for Cervical Ripening in Term Pregnancy." *FPIN's Clinical Inquiries*, February 1, 2006.

Wagner, Marsden, M.D. "Cytotec Induction and Off-Label Use." *Midwifery Today*, 2003.

Wagner, Marsden, M.D. "Misoprostol: More on the Dangers of Cytotec." *Midwifery Today*, 1999.

"What Is a Doula?" *DONA International*, 2005.

"What Is Placenta Calcification?" *The Labor of Love*, n.d.

"What Is the Birth Center Experience?" *The Birth Center Experience*, n.d.

CHAPTER 10: BRINGING UP BABY

Frost, Robert. "Stopping by Woods on a Snowy Evening." *The Poetry of Robert Frost*, 1923.

Turner, Tina. "What's Love Got to Do With It?" by Terry Britten and Graham Lyle. *Private Dancer*. Capitol Records, 1984.

CHAPTER 11: TO VACCINATE OR NOT TO VACCINATE

Barrett, Stephen, M.D. "Lancet Retracts Wakefield Paper." *Autism Watch,* May 29, 2010.

"Chickenpox and Pregnancy." *Centers for Disease Control and Prevention*, September 9, 2014.

"Common Ingredients in U.S. Licensed Vaccines." *U.S. Food and Drug Administration*, May 1, 2014.

Culp-Ressler, Tara. "The Anti-Vaccine Conspiracy Theory That Slips Under The Radar." *Think Progress*, February 11, 2015.

Deer, Brian. "Revealed: The MMR research scandal." *The Sunday Times* (London), Feb 24, 2004.

"The DTaP Vaccine." *Baby Center*, February 2015.

The Editors of The Lancet. "Retraction—Ileal-lymphoid-nodular Hyperplasia, Non-specific Colitis, and Pervasive Developmental Disorder in Children." *The Lancet,* 2010.

"11 Things More Likely to Happen than Winning the Powerball Jackpot." *NBC News*, November 28, 2011.

Fischer, T.K., C. Vibaud, U. Parashar, M. Malek, C. Steiner, R. Glass, and L. Simonsen. "Hospitalizations and Deaths from Diarrhea and Rotavirus among Children." *National Center for Biotechnology Information* (U.S. National Library of Medicine), March 6, 2007. *The Journal of Infectious Diseases* 195.8 (2007): 1117–25.

"Frequently Asked Questions about Measles in the U.S." *Centers for Disease Control and Prevention*, January 29, 2015.

Garrey, Sascha. "Opting-Out Of Vaccines; Dipping Below Herd Immunity." *WBUR'S Common Health*, August 22, 2013.

Godlee, Fiona, Jane Smith, and Harvey Marcovitch, ed. "Wakefield's Article Linking MMR Vaccine and Autism Was Fraudulent." *BMJ*, January 6, 2011.

Gupta, Rupal Christine, ed. "Whooping Cough (Pertussis)." *KidsHealth*, February 1, 2015.

Haelle, Tara. "'There Are Just Too Many Shots'... and Other Reasons Some Parents Don't Want to Vaccinate." *Parents,* October 2015.

Hunter, Wendy, M.D. "8 Simple Rules for Raising a Healthy Kid." *Parents,* January 2016

Koplow, David A. *Smallpox: The Fight to Eradicate a Global Scourge.* University of California Press, 2003.

"The Lancet Retracts Andrew Wakefield's Article." *Science Based Medicine*, February 3, 2010.

MacDonald, Fiona. "The U.S. Is in the Middle of Its Biggest Measles Outbreak This Year." *ScienceAlert*, July 12, 2016.

"Measles (Rubeola)." *Centers for Disease Control and Prevention*, February 13, 2015.

"Measles Cases and Outbreaks." *Centers for Disease Control and Prevention*, November 18, 2015.

"Measles Led to Death of Clallam Co. Woman; First in U.S. in a Dozen Years." *Department of Health Washington*, July 2, 2015.

"Measles—United States, 2011." *Centers for Disease Control and Prevention*, April 20, 2012.

Mercola, Joseph. "The Case Against Aluminum in Vaccines." *Mercola.com,* March 31, 2015.

Nelson, Bryan. "8 Deadly Diseases Cured by Modern Science." *Mother Nature Network*, August 20, 2013.

"New Meta-analysis Confirms: No Association between Vaccines and Autism." *Autism Speaks*, May 19, 2014.

Nierenburg, Carie. "Whooping Cough Outbreak: How Effective Is the Vaccine?" *Live Science*, January 13, 2016.

"Pertussis Cases by Year (1922–2014)." *Centers for Disease Control and Prevention*, September 8, 2015.

"Pertussis: Questions and Answers." *Immunization Action Coalition,* 1983.

"Possible Side-effects from Vaccines." Centers for Disease Control and Prevention, n.d.

"Pregnancy: Your Baby's First Hours of Life." *Women's Health*, September 27, 2010.

Raines, Katie. "Formaldehyde: A Poison and Carcinogen Used in Vaccines." *Health Impact News*, November 10, 2015.

"Smallpox." *Web Archive Wayback Machine*, June 11, 2003.

Tomljenovic, L., and C.A. Shaw. "Aluminum Vaccine Adjuvants: Are They Safe?" *National Center for Biotechnology Information* (U.S. National Library of Medicine), 2011.

"Useless Facts—Statistics 2." *Brain of Brian*, n.d.

"Vaccine Adjuvants." *Centers for Disease Control and Prevention*, September 12, 2016.

"Vaccine and Immunization: Whooping Cough and the Vaccine (Shot) to Prevent It." *Centers for Disease Control and Prevention*, August 14, 2015.

"Vaccine Excipient and Media Summary." *Epidimiology and Prevention of Vaccine-Preventable Diseases, 13th Edition*, February 2015.

"Vaccine Timeline: Historic Dates and Events Related to Vaccines and Immunization." *Immunize*, 2013.

"Vaccines Do Not Cause Autism." *Centers for Disease Control and Prevention*, October 27, 2015.

Wakefield, A.J., S.H. Murch, A. Anthony, J. Linell, D. M. Casson, M. Malik, M. Berelowitz, A. P. Dhillon, M. A. Thompson, P. Harvey, A. Valentine, S. E. Davies, and J. A. Walker-Smith. "Ileal-lymphoid-nodular Hyperplasia, Non-specific Colitis, and Pervasive Developmental Disorder in Children." *The Lancet* 352.9123 (1998): 234–35.

W., Todd. "Demystifying Vaccine Ingredients — Formaldehyde." *Harpocrates Speaks*, April 5, 2012.

CHAPTER 12: SICK IS A FOUR-LETTER WORD

"Acetaminophen Linked to Asthma in New Report." *NBC News*, November 7, 2011.

Adhisivam, B. "Is Gripe Water Baby-Friendly?" *Journal of Pharmacology & Pharmacotherapeutics*, April 2012.

Bayless, Kate. "Your No-Panic Guide to Fever." *Parents,* December 2015.

Cara, Ed. "Ibuprofen vs. Acetaminophen: How Different Are They Really?" *Medical Daily*, January 5, 2016.

Cohen, Scott W. *Eat, Sleep, Poop: A Common Sense Guide to Your Baby's First Year.* New York: Scribner, 2010.

"Cradle Cap." *Mayo Clinic Organization*, November 12, 2015.

"¿Cuándo Debe Llamar al Pediatra Debido a Una Fiebre?" *HealthyChildren.org*, May 1, 2016.

"Ear Infections." *Health CVS*, December 15, 2015.

"ELDERBERRY: Uses, Side Effects, Interactions and Warnings." *WebMD*, n.d.

Essential Oils Natural Remedies: The Complete A–Z Reference of Essential Oils for Health and Healing. Berkeley, CA: Althea Press, 2015.

"Fever without Fear: Information for Parents." *Healthy Children*, April 22, 2016.

"Getting Smart About Antibiotics." *Health*, September 2016.

Holman, Tayla, and Erica Roth. "Treating Acid Reflux in Infants." *Healthline*, May 5, 2015.

"How to Measure Fever with Different Thermometers." *Parents*, n.d.

Hum, Martin. "Vanquishing Viruses – 10 Natural Antiviral Remedies." *ION*, Spring 2004.

Hunter, Wendy, M.D. "8 Simple Rules for Raising a Healthy Kid." *Parents*, January 2016.

Landau, Meryl Davids. "Baby-Safe Alternative Medicine." *Parenting*, n.d.

Landau, Meryl Davids. "14 Natural Health Remedies for Children." *Parents*, May 2008.

Marquez, Jennifer Rainey. "Cold Comfort." *Parents,* January 2016.

"MULLEIN: Uses, Side Effects, Interactions and Warnings." *WebMD*, n.d.

Neitz, Katie McDonald. "What to Do When Baby Gets Sick: 7 Solutions." *Parents*, n.d.

Reisser, Paul C. *Focus on the Family Complete Guide to Baby & Child Care: From Pre-Birth through the Teen Years.* Wheaton, IL: Tyndale House, 2007.

Rowlands, Letitia. "Why Drinking Water Can Be Deadly for Babies." *Essential Baby*, May 20, 2015.

Sears, William, M.D. "Dr. Sears: Guide to the Top 7 Infant Illnesses." *Parenting*, n.d.

"Signs and Symptoms of Fever." *HealthyChildren.org*, November 21, 2015.

Stoppard, Miriam. "Medical Index." *New Babycare*, 2007.

"A Warning about Vicks VapoRub." *Parenting*, 2011.

Watson, Stephanie, and Rena Goldman. "Is It a Cold or the Flu?" *Healthline*, March 23, 2015.

Whiteman, Honor. "Antibiotic Resistance: How Has It Become a Global Threat to Public Health?" *Medical News Today*, September 10, 2014.

CHAPTER 13: BREASTFEEDING SUCKS

Alperin, Tracey. "Breastfeeding Reactions." *Mommy-life, Doula, Wife,* August 8, 2014.

Antonow-Schlorkea, Iwa, Matthias Schwaba, Laura Coxb, Kristina Stuchlika, Otto W. Wittea, Peter W. Nathanielszc, and Thomas J. McDonald. "Vulnerability of the Fetal Primate Brain to Moderate Reduction in Maternal Global Nutrient Availability." *PNAS*, December 21, 2010.

"Baby Formula Has Such a Bad Rap, Moms Are Buying Contaminated Breast Milk Online." *Yahoo News*, April 6, 2015.

BabyCenter Medical Advisory Board, ed. "How Breastfeeding Benefits You and Your Baby." *BabyCenter*, n.d.

Ballard, Olivia, and Ardythe L. Morrow. "Human Milk Composition: Nutrients and Bioactive Factors." *Pediatric Clinics of North America*, February 6, 2013.

"Benefits of Breastmilk." *Ask Dr Sears*, n.d.

Ben-Joseph, Elana Pearl. "Breastfeeding vs. Formula Feeding." *KidsHealth*, February 1, 2015.

Bonyata, Kelly, IBCLC. "Breastfeeding and Alcohol." *Kelly Mom*, March 3, 2016.

"Breast Pumping Tips." *Ask Dr Sears*, August 12, 2013.

"Breastfeeding and Fertility." *Ask Dr Sears,* August 12, 2013.

Brigham and Women's Hospital. "Breastfeeding associated with better brain development, neurocognitive outcomes." *ScienceDaily.* July 29, 2016.

Brody, Jane E. "The Ideal and the Real of Breast-Feeding." *The New York Times*, July 23, 2012.

Cohen, Scott W. *Eat, Sleep, Poop: A Common Sense Guide to Your Baby's First Year.* New York: Scribner, 2010.

Corleone, Jill, RDN, LD. "Soy Formula vs. Lactose-Free Formula." *LIVESTRONG.COM*, July 6, 2015.

Dermer, Alicia, M.D., IBCLC. "A Well-Kept Secret: Breastfeeding's Benefits to Mothers." *La Leche League International,* n.d. From: *NEW BEGINNINGS* 18.4 (2001): n.p.

Dewar, Gwen, Ph.D. "Nutrients and Calories in Breast Milk: A Guide for the Science-Minded." *Parenting Science,* 2008.

Dietz, William H., M.D., Ph.D. "Breastfeeding May Help Prevent Childhood Overweight." *JAMA Network*, May 16, 2001.

"Does Breastfeeding Reduce the Risk of Allergies?" *InteliHealth*, n.d.

Eidelman, Arthur I., M.D., and Richard Schanler, M.D. "Breastfeeding and the Use of Human Milk." *Pediatrics,* 2012.

Elding, Craig. "Formula vs Breastfeeding." *The Health Cloud,* August 21, 2013.

"Exclusive Breastfeeding to Reduce the Risk of Childhood Overweight and Obesity." *World Health Organization*, September 2014.

Fisher, Denise. "Social Drugs and Breastfeeding." *Health E-Learning*, n.d.

Garber, Megan. "A Brief History of Breast Pumps." *The Atlantic*, October 21, 2013.

Gilman, Charlotte Perkins. *The Yellow Wallpaper and Other Stories.* Mineola, NY: Dover Publications, 1997.

Hale, Thomas Wright, Ph.D., and Hilary E. Rowe, PharmD. *Medications and Mothers' Milk.* Amarillo, TX: Hale Pub., 2010.

Hamm, Trent. "How Much Money Does Breastfeeding Really Save?" *The Simple Dollar*, October 12, 2013.

Hauck, Fern R., John M.D. Thompson, Kawai O. Tanabe, Rachel Y. Moon, and Mechtild M. Vennemann. "Breastfeeding and Reduced Risk of

Sudden Infant Death Syndrome: A Meta-analysis." *Pediatrics*, June 2011.

Hope, Jenny. "Call for U-turn on When to Wean Baby after Warnings That Exclusively Breast-feeding for Six Months 'Causes Allergies'. *Daily Mail*, January 14, 2011.

Horwood, L. John, and David M. Fergusson. "Breastfeeding and Later Cognitive and Academic Outcomes." *Pediatrics* 101.1 (1998): n.p.

Huotari, Carol. "Alcohol and Motherhood." *La Leche League International*, October 14, 2007. From: *LEAVEN* 33.2 (1997): n.p.

Jacobson, Hilary. "Beer as a Galactagogue—A Brief History." *A Lactogenic Diet*, October 13, 2011.

James, Maia. "HiPP Versus Holle: Which Formula?" *Gimme the Good Stuff*, February 23, 2016.

James, Maia. "Safe Infant Formula Guide." *Gimme the Good Stuff*, March 2015.

Jones, Wendy, Ph.D., MRPharmS. "Alcohol and Breastfeeding." *The Breastfeeding Network,* October 2012.

Kraft, Sy. "Oral Thrush In Babies: Causes, Symptoms and Treatments." *Medical News Today*, n.d.

Lepore, Jill. "Baby Food: If Breast Is Best, Why Are Women Bottling Their Milk?" *New Yorker*, January 19, 2009.

Levine, Hallie. "Bone Up Your Bones: The Hormone Factor." *Health Magazine,* May 2016.

MacDonald, Elizabeth. "Baby Formula: How to Make the Best Decision." *My Baby's Heartbeat Bear,* September 30, 2016.

Marks, V., and J.W. Wright. "Endocrinological and Metabolic Effects of Alcohol." *National Center for Biotechnology Information* (U.S. National Library of Medicine), n.d. Originally published in *Proceedings of the Royal Society of Medicine* 70.5 (1977): 337–344.

Mazumdar, Madhumita Das, M.D. "Age of Onset of Menopause." *Gynaeonline,* n.d.

Mennella, Julie A., Ph.D. "Regulation of Milk Intake After Exposure to Alcohol in Mothers' Milk." *National Center for Biotechnology Information* (U.S. National Library of Medicine), n.d. Originally published in *Alcoholism Clinical & Experimental Research* 25.4 (2001): 590–593.

Mennella, Julie A., Ph.D., and Gary K. Beauchamp, Ph.D. "The Transfer of Alcohol to Human Milk—Effects on Flavor and the Infant's Behavior.*" The New English Journal of Medicine* 325.14 (1991): 981–985.

Mohrbacher, Nancy, and Julie Stock. *The Breastfeeding Answer Book.* Schaumburg, IL: La Leche League International, 1997.

Morrisey, Tracey Egan. "The Pressure to Breastfeed Is Getting Out of Hand." *Jezebel,* July 8, 2012.

Newman, Jack, Ph.D. *More Breastfeeding Myths.* n.d.

Nordqvist, Christian. "Mastitis: Causes, Symptoms and Treatments." *Medical News Today,* September 30, 2015.

O'Connor, Mary, M.D. MPH. "Breastfeeding & Drugs: Alcohol." *Breastfeeding Basics,* 1998.

Reinberg, Steven. "Breast-feeding May Shield Against Sudden Infant Death Syndrome." *U.S. News,* June 13, 2011.

Rosin, Hanna. "The Case Against Breast-Feeding." *The Atlantic,* April 1, 2009.

Saslow, Debbie, Ph.D. "Can Breastfeeding Lower Breast Cancer Risk?" *American Cancer Society – Expert Voices Blog,* May 7, 2013.

Sundstrum, Kelly. "Think You Can't Get Pregnant While Breastfeeding? Think Again!" *Parenting,* n.d.

"Taurine, Energy Drinks and Bull Sperm: Ten Things to Know." *Fooducate,* July 2012.

"Top Tips from Moms Who Pump." *BabyCenter,* n.d.

Vallaeys, Charlotte. "How To Find the Safest Organic Infant Formula." *Cornucopia Institute,* December 20, 2013.

Vennemann, M.M., T. Bajanowski, B. Brinkmann, G. Jorch, K. Yücesan, C. Sauerland, and E.A. Mitchell. "Does Breastfeeding Reduce the Risk of Sudden Infant Death Syndrome?" *Pediatrics* 123.3 (2009): n.p.

"Vitamin D Supplementation." *Centers for Disease Control and Prevention,* June 17, 2015.

Wiessinger, Diane, and Diana West. *The Womanly Art of Breastfeeding.* New York, NY: Plume, 1997.

"Yeast Infections or Thrush." *Breastfeeding Basics,* September 17, 2015.

Zeretzke, Karen. "Yeast Infections and the Breastfeeding Family: Helping Mothers Find Relief for Symptoms and Treatment for the Infection Preserves the Breastfeeding Relationship." *La Leche League International*, August 29, 2006. From: *LEAVEN* 34.5 (1998): 91–96.

CHAPTER 14: *THE BABY, THE BOSS, THE HOME, & YOUR LOVER*

Adams, Richard. "Having a Working Mother Works for Daughters." *The Guardian*, June 24, 2015.

"Balance Work and Family." *Pew Social Trends*, March 13, 2013.

Capetta, Amy. "Going Back to Work After Baby." *Parents*, n.d.

Cohn, D'Vera, Gretchen Livingston, and Wendy Wang. "After Decades of Decline, A Rise in Stay-at-Home Mothers." *Pew Social Trends*, April 8, 2014.

The Council of Economic Advisers, comp. "Nine Facts About American Families and Work." *Executive Office of the President of the United States,* June 2014.

"Family and Medical Leave Act." *National Partnership for Women & Families*, n.d.

Hall, Katy. "Paid Parental Leave: U.S. vs. The World (INFOGRAPHIC)." *The Huffington Post*, April 2, 2013.

"The Harried Life of the Working Mother." *Pew Social Trends*, October 1, 2009.

Manca, Giuliana. "Countries With Best Maternity Leave Benefits." *The Epoch Times*, April 28, 2016.

McGinn, Kathleen L., Mayra Ruiz Castro, and Elizabeth Long Lingo. "Mums the Word! Cross-national Effects of Maternal Employment on Gender Inequalities at Work and at Home." *Harvard Business School*, 2015.

National Partnership for Women & Families, comp. "State Paid Family Leave Insurance Laws." *State Paid Family Leave Insurance Laws,* February 2015.

Parker, Kim, and Wendy Wang. "Modern Parenthood: Roles of Moms and Dads Converge as They Balance Work and Family." *Pew Social Trends*, March 14, 2013.

Patel, Arti. "Worst And Best Countries For Maternity Leave." *The Huffington Post*, May 22, 2012.

Ramnarace, Cynthia. "Maternity Leave and Benefits Around the World." *The Bump*, n.d.

"Statistics: Who Is Happier – Working Moms or Stay at Home Moms?" *Proud Working Mom*, February 4, 2015.

CHAPTER 15: DOGGED MOMMY GUILT

Nirvana. "Dumb," by Kurt Cobain. *In Utero.* DGC, 1993.

AFTERWORD: POSTPARTUM REFLECTIONS

Guido, Maria. "First Baby Destroys Happiness Worse Than Divorce Or Death, Says Science." *Scary Mommy*, n.d.

Turgeon, Heather, MFT, and Julie Wright, MFT. *The Happy Sleeper: The Science-backed Guide To Helping Your Baby Get a Good Night's Sleep—Newborn to School Age.* New York, NY: TarcherPerigee, 2014.

Wolf, Naomi. *Misconceptions: Truth, Lies, and the Unexpected on the Journey to Motherhood.* New York: Doubleday, 2001.